CW00546200

Liberate Your R

86 articles about Reiki.

One inspiring vision.

by Taggart King

*To Dear Sophia,
With Reiki hugs!*

www.reiki-evolution.co.uk
taggart@reiki-evolution.co.uk

ISBN 978-0-9563168-9-9

My manifesto for Reiki tolerance 8

THE 10 RULES OF REIKI 13

(1) Reiki is all about you..14
(2) Base your practice on the precepts 16
(3) Practise mindfulness 20
(4) Work on yourself daily 24
(5) Commitment is the key 28
(6) Don't try too hard...31
(7) You don't need to be perfect 36
(8) Don't keep trying to puzzle out 'why' 40
(9) Trust your intuition 44
(10) Ignore silly rules and restrictions..................................46
The Ten Rules of Reiki in a few sentences 50

FUNDAMENTALS 51

Back to Basics: Reiki First Degree 52
The Precepts 63
Mindfulness and Compassion 67
How to start a Reiki treatment..71
What hand positions should I use? 75
How long should I spend in each hand position? 78
Do I need to keep at least one hand on a person when I treat
them? 81
Reiki Sensations 84
Treating both sides: is this necessary?..................................91
What if I get it wrong?..95
Declutter your treatment rituals...101
Reiki treatments and winning the lottery 106
Reiki is not all fluffy bunnies! 109
The Kaizen of Reiki 113
Get out of the way! 122
Reiki advice from Bruce Lee: Be like water 126
Simple energy exercises to get the energy flowing 129
The simplest self-treatment meditation ever! 133
Intuitive self-healing meditation 136
Mikao Usui's original self-treatment meditation.................139
Intuitive hands-on self-treatment method 142
The simplest hands-on self-treatment method ever 145

THE "21 DAY" THING 146
YOUR 10 DAY REIKI CHALLENGE: THE "RELEASING EXERCISE" 150
USING REIKI FOR ANXIETY 157
USING REIKI FOR STRESS.. 160
CAN YOU SEND DISTANT HEALING AT REIKI FIRST DEGREE? 163
RESTRICTIONS ON REIKI 166
INTELLIGENT ENERGY? 174

DEVELOPING YOUR REIKI 180

BACK TO BASICS: REIKI SECOND DEGREE 181
THE BREATH OF EARTH AND HEAVEN 191
DO I ALWAYS HAVE TO USE THE SYMBOLS? 195
REIKI SYMBOLS, ATTUNEMENTS AND BEYOND.............................. 198
SIMPLICITY AND SANDWICHES 204
A SIMPLE WAY WITH SYMBOLS 209
WERE YOU TAUGHT THE CORRECT "POWER" SYMBOL: VARIATIONS ON
CKR... 213
SOME HERESY ABOUT REIKI SYMBOLS 217
LET'S EXPLORE SOME NON-REIKI SYMBOLS 221
CREATE YOUR OWN BESPOKE REIKI SYMBOLS 224
CREATE A BESPOKE REIKI SYMBOL FOR YOUR CLIENT 228
THE SIMPLEST DISTANT HEALING METHOD EVER! 232
DISTANT HEALING WITH IMAGINED HAND POSITIONS 234
DISTANT HEALING WITH A LITTLE BIT OF RITUAL ATTACHED 236
DISTANT HEALING USING SOME SORT OF A PROP 240
DO I NEED PERMISSION TO SEND DISTANT HEALING? 242
SENDING REIKI DISTANT HEALING TO THE PAST 244
SENDING REIKI DISTANT HEALING TO THE FUTURE.......................... 246
DITCH THE DOGMA IN REIKI DISTANT HEALING 248
DISTANT HEALING, ONENESS AND MIKAO USUI'S ORIGINAL SYSTEM. 250
HSZSN BUT NOT AS YOU'VE SEEN IT BEFORE! 253
WORKING WITH INTUITION.. 256
YOU CAN BECOME MORE INTUITIVE WITH YOUR REIKI 262
DEVELOP YOUR REIKI INTUITION (PART I) 265
DEVELOP YOUR REIKI INTUITION (PART II)................................... 267
DEVELOP YOUR REIKI INTUITION (PART III) 269
DEVELOP YOUR REIKI INTUITION (PART IV) 273
THE IMPORTANCE OF INTENT 277
SCANNING AT A DISTANCE.. 281

REMOTE TREATMENTS 283
FENG SHUI YOUR REIKI 287
BEWARE REIKI "KNOW-IT-ALLS" 294

FOR MASTERS...298

DO ATTUNEMENTS ACTUALLY WORK? 299
BECOME A SUPER POWER REIKI MASTER IN JUST 48 HOURS? WHAT A
JOKE! 303
THE FOUNDER OF WESTERN REIKI DID DISTANT ATTUNEMENTS! 306
ATTUNEMENTS, EMPOWERMENTS & THE REIKI CONTACT LENS
SCANDAL! 310
ADVICE FOR NEW REIKI TEACHERS 320
STRUCTURING YOUR REIKI COURSE 324
REIKI TEACHING: EXPLAIN, GUIDE AND REVIEW 328
REIKI TEACHING: TELL THEM, TELL THEM AND TELL THEM 332
REIKI TEACHING: YOUR COURSE MATERIALS 337
REIKI TEACHING: SUPPORTING YOUR STUDENTS 342
REIKI TEACHING: WHAT ARE YOUR GOALS? 347
REIKI TEACHING: USING LEARNING PREFERENCES 352
REIKI TEACHING: USING THE RIGHT 4MAT 358
HOW REIKI EVOLUTION CAN HELP YOU WITH YOUR REIKI COURSES ..363

About this book

This book contains most of the Reiki articles that I have written over the last 20 years. You'll find over 80 of them and they deal with all aspects of practising this beautiful and simple system.

I have called this collection "Liberate your Reiki!" and I hope you will find running through these articles a vision of Reiki as a simple and powerful self-development tool and treatment method, free from the clutter, busyness and dogma of Western Reiki practice.

I root my vision of Reiki in the original practices of Mikao Usui, Reiki's founder, and I try to emphasise the need for simplicity, flexibility, personal dedication and commitment in obtaining the many benefits that are available to the student through Reiki.

The articles I have written fall comfortably into three themes:

1. Reiki fundamentals
2. Developing yourself further
3. Help for Reiki Master Teachers

Though you could see the first two categories as corresponding to the two Reiki levels (First Degree and Second Degree), I think that all the articles there should be of interest to and of benefit to all Reiki people at whatever Reiki level.

How to use this book

Don't read the whole book all in one go. Take your time to work through the essays; there's no rush!

Read an essay or two every day and ponder its contents. Think about your own practice of Reiki and whether what you have read has helped in some way:

- Have some of your questions been answered?
- Do you now have further questions?
- Are you prompted to try something new or practise something in a different way?
- Are you prompted to add something to your practice?
- Are you prompted to eliminate something from your practice?

I want you to scribble in this book!

This is a practical workbook, so I want to see you writing in it. Write in it anywhere: underline or circle things, put exclamation marks, arrows and asterisks, jot in the margins, write "NO!!!", write "ABSOLUTELY YES!!", write "NONSENSE!!", write "THIS IS SO TRUE!!".

I hope that these articles make a difference to you and that your practice of Reiki is enhanced as a result.

With best wishes,

Taggart King
Reiki Evolution
www.reiki-evolution.co.uk

My manifesto for Reiki tolerance

Honouring all the flavours of Reiki

The lovely thing about Reiki is that there are so many styles, so many different ways of working with the energy. Various people on the Internet have tried to compile lists of the different versions, and I think the total runs to a hundred or more.

Reiki seems to work as an effortless 'carrier', rather like a radio station and transmitter that you can play endless different songs through, but you need the underlying radio waves before the songs can be played.

Reiki is like those radio waves: a carrier that supports very many different ways of working.

What Reiki song do you sing?

Is it Karuna Reiki or Seichem, is it Reiki Tummo or Celtic Reiki or 'Traditional Usui' (in all its sub-flavours), is your song Jikiden or Raku Kei?

Or maybe it's Rainbow Reiki or Lightarian Reiki, Violet Flame or Usui-do.

Some systems use a few different symbols, some use *loads* of symbols, some are structured, others are more 'content free'; Reiki accommodates them all.

And it is true that some people will be attracted to a particular approach over another because everyone is different and one approach may feel more 'right' to one person than another.

I like to get back to the historical roots of things

To my eternal shame, I suppose, I am into folk music [there, I have said it: I like folk music!]. I play the five-string banjo.

But rather than playing Bluegrass music, which came into being in the 1950s, I prefer to play 'clawhammer' style banjo, which takes you back to the very beginnings of 'Old Time' music when the syncopated 'slave style' of playing blended with immigrants' Irish and English tunes.

It feels right to me to play in a way that is authentic and 'original', so far as it is possible to recreate that style.

I also dabble with the 'Anglo' concertina and my preference is to get back to playing the 'original' English Anglo concertina style, so far as it is possible to glean what that was.

So it's not surprising, then, that when I became involved in Reiki I was attracted to what was known about the form of Reiki that Usui Sensei was teaching in the 1920s in Japan, rather than the later styles that had developed and changed and mutated after the time of Mrs Takata.

Discovering Original Japanese Reiki

I was lucky enough to have been in the right place at the right time, and received a lot of guidance from people who brought me a lot closer to understanding what the original system was all about, and my "Reiki Evolution" courses are based on that principle: to practise Reiki, so far as it is possible or practical, in a way that comes close to what we know that Usui was teaching to most of his students.

And for me that's the bee's knees, a wonderful way to practise that, *for me*, is much more fulfilling than the more standard 'Western-style' Reiki that I was first taught.

And we have taught many other Reiki people from a standard Western background who have found that the original system that we teach has many advantages.

There is no 'one true way'

But not everyone is attracted to that way of practising Reiki because everyone is different, of course, and what I want to make clear is that I do not believe that what I teach is the 'one true way', the Reiki that everyone should learn, better than everyone else's.

How arrogant and blinkered that would be, if I was to say such a thing.

I meet many lovely and open Reiki practitioners and teachers, who are happy and content to be practising Reiki in their unique way, and to accept that others can practise Reiki in their different way, and that's it's ok to differ. These are the Reiki people that I want to spend my time with: those who are open and content with the path that they are following, and who do not feel the need to look down their nose and impose their flavour and their rules on everyone else.

The curse of blinkered dogma

Sadly, there are some Reiki teachers out there who do actually believe that their way of teaching Reiki is the 'correct' way, that there is a 'correct' way to use the symbols, for example, and that if someone has been taught in a different way then they're wrong.

This is sad.

This is divisive.

There are even people who believe that an attunement needs to be carried out in a certain prescribed fashion in order to be 'correct', yet the attunements that Mrs Takata taught have evolved and changed endlessly in different lineages; some are almost unrecogniseable.

And do you know what? They all work fine.

So I think we should be wary of Reiki Masters, no matter how prominent they appear to be, who tell you that what you are doing is wrong or that you shouldn't do a particular thing: we are all on our journey with the energy, and our journey is our journey, leading us to practise in *our* way, not better, not worse, just different.

My belief

I believe that we should celebrate these differences, and be happy that there is infinite variety.

I believe that Reiki people should be free to find their own comfortable path with the energy, working in the way that suits them, rather than having to kow tow to the dogma and blinkered beliefs of another.

Over to you

So there you have it: my 'manifesto' for tolerance, acceptance, and mutual respect within Reiki.

I hope you agree with me.

The 10 Rules of Reiki

In this article I thought I would set down ten things that you can do – ten principles to take account of – to benefit your practice of Reiki. This is not something that has come from Japan, or from early practitioners of Reiki: it is just something that I have put together myself. I hope that this article will be of interest to people at all Reiki levels.

(1) Reiki is all about you

Although in many circles, Reiki is seen as basically a hands-on healing system, a complementary therapy, something that you do to other people, it hasn't always been like that and if your Reiki is mainly about working on other people then you really are missing out on a system that has the potential to transform your life in so many ways!

If we go back to the origins of the system and Mikao Usui's original teachings, treating other people didn't feature a great deal at all: it was all about working on yourself.

We know that the word "Reiki" wasn't used by Usui, and that he referred to his system as a "method to achieve personal perfection", so that gives us a big hint as to the main thrust of his system: working on ourselves.

And I know that most Reiki systems will include hands-on self-treatments, and the precepts will be referred to, but there's a lot more to Usui's system in terms of self-healing, and spirituality, and self-development, if we can embrace the original practices and make them the foundation of what we do with Reiki.

What I'm talking about here are daily energy exercises and some form of self-treatment, I'm talking about the practice of mindfulness, and an ongoing focus on Mikao Usui's original precepts. When taken together, these practices when carried out on a regular basis have the potential to make such a difference to people.

Interestingly, I have heard some people saying that it's a bit selfish to use Reiki on yourself, that you should be spending your time working on other people, and I don't agree with this of course: it seems a very strange belief to choose.

Firstly, by treating other people you are also benefiting from the energy that you are channelling, so there's no way of separating out the energy so that it's only benefiting the person you're working on, and ignoring you.

Secondly, if we are following the Reiki system, following the precepts that deal with compassion and honesty, then how can we neglect ourselves? How can we deliberately refuse to nurture ourselves, refuse to give ourselves that special space in which to heal and balance?

I know it can be scary sometimes having to deal what's holding us back in our lives, and change can be frightening, but it's only by striving to be the best person that we can be – by letting go of emotions that are stifling us, by allowing the energy to heal us on all levels – that we can truly help others in the most powerful and positive way, because we can then channel the energy from a place of composure and mindfulness, a still calm vessel for the energy, channelled by someone who is a living embodiment of the many blessings that Reiki can bring into our lives.

So be an advert for what Reiki can do for you: work on yourself, let go of anger and worry, embrace compassion and forgiveness for yourself and embody the benefits of this wonderful system.

(2) Base your practice on the precepts

It's interesting that whereas in the Judaeo-Christian tradition we are given a list of things that we shouldn't do: "thou shalt not kill" etc, in Buddhism, followers are given a list of precepts or rules to live by that seem to be framed in more of a positive way.

And in Mikao Usui's system, he also provided his students with a simple, or apparently simple, set of precepts to follow, which seemed to be a way of distilling the essence of Tendai Buddhist principles into a form that anyone could understand. His five precepts have a long history, coming from a Tendai sect of Shugendo that Usui was in contact with, and this is what they are:

Just for today
Do not anger
Do not worry
Be humble
Be honest in your dealings with people
Be compassionate to yourself and others

The most important precept

For me, the first phrase is the most important, the "just for today...".

For me, this encapsulates all that follows it.

"Just for today" means being in a mindful state, fully engaged in the moment. If you are fully engaged with the present moment then you are in a state that is free from anger and worry, which are based on either dwelling on the past or imagining the future.

So "Just for today" means being in a state that is free from anger and free from worry. We don't want to distract ourselves through fear and we can remind ourselves that all is illusion.

We can simply exist in the moment.

And in that mindful space, you have the room to be compassionate, compassionate and forgiving towards other people and compassionate and forgiving towards yourself, being mindful means being in a centred, nurturing space where you can embrace honesty (and being honest with yourself is as important as being honest towards others) a space where you can truly experience the many blessings that you have in your life.

It all stems from, "Just for today".

The very heart of Usui's system

These five precepts are at the very heart of Usui's system and it was said that as much spiritual development could come through following the precepts as could come through carrying out the energy work.

So how can we work with the precepts?

Well we need to remind ourselves of them on a regular basis, and some people will say them out loud each day, perhaps as part of their routine of daily energy exercises and meditations. Maybe you could recite them in your head.

But it's not enough to just know what they are: the precepts need to infiltrate themselves into our daily lives, our thoughts, feelings and our behaviour. And we can achieve this in a couple of ways…

Firstly, we can ponder a particular precept, examining it and how it might have affected our lives, had we lived our lives by that precept in the past. How would we have behaved in past situations, how would we have reacted differently, or dealt with people, if we had embodied that particular precept?

1. What would we have felt, what would be have been thinking in different past situations if we were living that precept fully?
2. How would things have gone differently or been better for us and maybe for other people?
3. How would that precept have affected your relationships or your priorities?

Do some mental 're-runs' of past events and see how they would have been different had you been following that precept.

Doing this can provide you with some useful insights into how a particular precept can make your life flow more smoothly.

Precepts rehearsal

Secondly, what you can do is to imagine some future situations or scenarios, events where, based on what you have discovered about your past, you can imagine things going differently in the future.

Bring to mind typical future events or scenes which would benefit from the use of that precept, and imagine yourself in that future situation, embodying that precept, and notice how that future event runs its course; notice the differences in the way that you think and feel, become aware of the ways that you are behaving and reacting differently, responding to people differently. Bring to mind clearly the new you who uses that precept as part of their daily life.

If you do this over a number of days, you will have a very clear idea of how the precepts could have changed past events in a positive way, and a solid understanding of how the precepts can be used by you in the future in different circumstances and events, how the precepts will work their way through your life, changing things for the better in many ways.

The precepts are something that we drip-feed into our daily lives, a work-in-progress where, over time, they become more and more a part of our basic blueprint.

We don't have to be perfect, though: we don't have to follow the precepts every waking moment and then beat ourselves up because we didn't achieve that. We are allowed to be human, we are allowed to not be perfect, which is all about embodying compassion and forgiveness for ourselves.

(3) Practise mindfulness

Although mindfulness is something that doesn't tend to turn up very often on most Reiki courses, it was actually a very important part of the system that Mikao was teaching, dovetailing with the precepts and the energy work to create a powerful method for self-healing and personal development.

And as you will have heard earlier, the practice of mindfulness is hidden in the Reiki precepts, hidden inside the phrase "just for today..." which for me is the most important part of the precepts: the phrase from which the other precepts flow.

So what is mindfulness?

Well mindfulness is a form of meditation that you can do anytime, anywhere.

You don't need to be sitting alone in a quiet room, setting aside time each day for your mindfulness practice: mindfulness is a meditation that can become part of your daily routines and activities. You can be mindful when you're doing the washing up, you can be mindful when you're eating your dinner, you can be mindful when you're typing on a keyboard or sipping cup of tea.

It is something that you can incorporate into your daily life as your daily life unfolds before you and it's not something that you need to set aside special time for, which makes it such a versatile way of meditating.

When you are mindful, you are consciously and fully aware of your thoughts and actions in the present moment, non-judgmentally, just existing in the moment, and in such a state you are free from thoughts of the past or the future, and free from the anger and the worry than can flow from such a dwelling on the past and the future.

By fully engaging with each moment, you are actually living your life, because all you have is this moment, this current awareness of the present: your life is a whole stream of present moments, and if you spend your time in the past and the future you are missing out on your life, because your life is here, now, not in the past, not in the future!

Find out more about mindfulness

The two books that I recommend about Mindfulness are both written by a Buddhist monk called Thich Nhat Hanh. The two books are "The Miracle of Mindfulness" and "Peace is every step: the path of mindfulness in everyday life".

I'd just like to read a small quote from Thich Nhat Hanh about mindfulness and washing dishes. Here goes:

"To my mind, the idea that doing dishes is unpleasant can occur only when you aren't doing them. Once you are standing in front of the sink with your sleeves rolled up and your hands in the warm water, it is really quite pleasant. I enjoy taking my time with each dish, being fully aware of the dish, the water, and each movement of my hands. I know that if I hurry in order to eat dessert sooner, the time of washing dishes will be unpleasant and not worth living. That would be a pity, for each minute, each second of life is a miracle. The dishes themselves and that fact that I am here washing them are miracles!"

So mindfulness is all about being fully aware of yourself, other people and your surroundings in the moment, focusing your awareness on each moment as it unfolds. And by doing that, you can savour each experience as it appears.

Getting started with Reiki mindfulness

Now obviously, when you start to practise mindfulness you are only going to gain little glimpses of that lovely 'in the moment' state, before your mind drags itself off to think about the past and the future, taking you away from your actual existence, and you need to be forgiving and compassionate.

This is a new way of doing things and it will take a while before your mind starts to understand how to do mindfulness consistently. Mindfulness is a work-in-progress and you'll find that over time those little glimpses of being 'in the moment' occur more frequently, you may find that occasionally you bliss out on some lovely mindful moments, and these moments, these glimpses, will build over time and become just a normal way of existing for you.

If your mind wanders, just gently bring your attention back to what you were doing, what you were experiencing.

There's no harm done.

Mindfulness lives in your Reiki practice already

You might be surprised to find that mindfulness is an integral part of your practice of Reiki.

When you're treating someone and you're in that lovely, merged state, blessed out on the energy, you're being mindful, just there in the moment, with the energy and the recipient, no expectations: that's mindfulness.

When you're sending distant healing, you've set your intent, maybe you've visualised something and you're just there, letting it happen, no thoughts of the past or future, just there with the energy: that's mindfulness.

So your mindfulness practice in your daily life – when doing the washing up, when eating a sandwich – will benefit your experience of mindfulness when using Reiki, and your experience of mindfulness when treating someone, or self-treating, or sending distant healing, will help you to experience mindfulness more easily during your everyday life.

You are training your mind, over time, to approach things in a different way, and your mind will learn what to do.

(4) Work on yourself daily

To get the most out of your Reiki, you need to have a regular practice of using the energy on yourself.

You're not going to gain the greatest benefits from this wonderful system that we all have if you just pick up Reiki once in a while, do something with it, and then put it down again for whatever period. So if you are looking for consistent benefits through Reiki then you need to have a consistent practice.

The precepts start by saying "just for today…" and we can extend that by saying, "Just for today I will do something with my Reiki".

And you can manage that; everyone can.

Everyone can make some time for Reiki each day because it doesn't have to be hours and hours and hours' worth. Do something for just 10 minutes: you have ten minutes. Do something for 20 minutes. And if you don't have 10 minutes then get up 10 minutes earlier in the morning: problem solved.

Everyone can find a way of doing something with their Reiki today, and we don't have to concern ourselves about tomorrow: tomorrow is another day. Tomorrow we'll start with "just for today I can do something with my Reiki", and we can find some time.

What could you do with your Reiki today?

Perhaps you're giving someone a full treatment, or perhaps you'll give someone a short blast of Reiki in your lunch-break: when you use Reiki on another person, you are gaining some benefit for yourself through channelling the energy. It doesn't pass through you without doing good things for you, and you'll be familiar with that lovely, chilled state that you experience as you get to the end of a Reiki session with someone else, almost as if you gain as much benefit as the person who's receiving!

Maybe someone has a bad back or a headache or an aching wrist: give them a short blast and snatch a little blissed-out-ness for yourself!

Can you take ten minutes in a lunch-break to become still and send some distant healing? That would be a lovely way to unwind and recharge your batteries half way through the day, while benefiting someone else at the same time.

Ten minutes of mindfulness and bathing in the energy at the same time.

Work on yourself in some way

You will have been taught a self-treatment method or methods, so use one on yourself, even if it's just for 10 minutes: you could just treat your shoulders, or rest your hands on your heart and solar plexus, which is a lovely way to experience the energy.

Have you tried that as a way of going off to sleep? The heat from your hands can be incredible sometimes, penetrating so deeply.

Take 10 minutes to do that for yourself, or maybe 15 minutes. Just drift with the energy as it flows. And of course you can do this for yourself whenever you're sitting down: do you sit at your desk reading something during your day: give yourself some Reiki as you do that.

Do you watch television? Reiki yourself as you do that and you might find that you start to drift off; that soap opera wasn't worth watching anyway! Preparing food... turn on your Reiki and channel it into what you're preparing: flood the kitchen with Reiki.

And you might be surprised how Reiki can turn itself on and flow when you're doing other things, particularly if you have some sort of a meditative practice that isn't Reiki: well, Reiki doesn't mind: it will turn itself on and click in, following your focus when you're doing any sort of meditation.

If you practise yoga or tai chi or chi kung:, Reiki will be there, being guided and moulded by your movements and visualisations, flowing and balancing and doing you good.

Build momentum

What's important here is the cumulative effect of using Reiki on yourself regularly, building momentum, small change building on previous small changes, taking you in the right direction for you.

Far better to do a bit each day than nothing for days and then doing a great big, long Reiki marathon on a weekend. That would be a wonderful experience, of course, and I'm not saying that you shouldn't do a mega Reiki session of you can, but make Reiki a regular part of your daily routine and you will be amazed by the benefits that this will bring you... remembering, of course, that you shouldn't beat yourself up if you don't manage to use Reiki every day.

Everything better than nothing is success and when we practise Reiki we embrace compassion and forgiveness, including forgiving ourselves for not being perfect, which of course we don't need to be in order to gain tremendous benefits from this simple spiritual system.

(5) Commitment is the key

There are spectacular benefits to be enjoyed through I've already spoken about the benefits that can come through the regular practise of Reiki, making working with the energy a regular part of your routine, trying to use the energy in some way each day.

The benefits of Reiki build up cumulatively, and sporadic and irregular practice won't be as effective in bringing you the very best that is possible for you through your Reiki.

Like many things, you'll get out of your Reiki what you are prepared to put into it, and Reiki deserves a little of your time each day. If you plug away, inch by inch, a few simple practices, a few simple routines, and make them a regular part of your daily and weekly routine, like brushing your teeth and brushing your hair – which you always make time for – then you'll get the very best out of your Reiki.

And once you have established your routine with Reiki it'll seem strange when you aren't doing your daily self-treatment or energy exercises, or distant healing. It doesn't take very long before your routine can just become part of who you are and it'll be difficult to avoid using your Reiki in some way.

So how do we commit to Reiki?

How do we make that decision, that final decision that cuts away all other possibilities?

Well I don't think you need to make such a decision. You just need to focus on today, and do something with your Reiki today, and that's all. And when the next day arrives, you repeat the process, doing something with your Reiki today.

One day at a time.

But there is something that you can do that can help you ease into your Reiki routine: visualise yourself doing what you intend to do.

Get yourself into a nice comfortable position and take a few deep breaths, perhaps do a bit of a self-treatment or part of hatsurei ho, to get the energy flowing, and imagine yourself doing what you plan to do: imagine yourself sitting down at lunchtime to do 10 minutes of distant healing, bring to mind how it will feel to send 15 minutes on a park bench just bringing the energy into your tanden and then flooding the energy out to the universe.

See yourself sitting on your sofa, blessed out for a while with an impromptu Reiki session, imagine yourself drifting off to sleep with your hands on your heart and solar plexus. See yourself doing these things as if you were watching yourself on a video, imagine how these things will feel, notice how you look and how your body seems so relaxed as you use your Reiki.

Imagine the benefits of doing this and see yourself experiencing those positive changes in the way that you behave and respond, those changes in the way that you feel about yourself and other people, changes in the way that you think. Just notice all those positive changes that come through your Reiki practice.

What you are doing here is mentally rehearsing what you days ahead, what your week ahead, will be like, and you are programming your mind to make these things happen, each day, to bring them to mind to remind you, to make them a priority.

Do this regularly and you'll be amazed by how simple it can be to ease into a really good routine with your Reiki.

(6) Don't try too hard

While we do need to commit ourselves and work with the energy regularly if we are to gain the greatest benefit through our connection to Reiki, working with mindfulness, focusing on the precepts and doing self treatments and other energy exercises as we can during our week, we also need to make sure that we aren't trying too hard at all this: it's supposed to be an enjoyable journey, not a big hard slog!

So we shouldn't take ourselves or our practice too seriously: Reiki is best enjoyed in a light-hearted fashion, in a gentle and laid-back way... not in a fists-clenched, furrowed-brow, tense 'read for a lot of hard work' sort of way.

We don't fore Reiki when we treat other people or when we work on ourselves and we shouldn't force a severe Reiki practice on ourselves either. That just wouldn't work: we should be doing our Reiki out of love, compassion, because we enjoy it.

Reiki is rather like a flowing stream and we're rather like a rough rock sitting in that stream.

The rock will become smooth over time but we can't force the river: the river flows at its own pace, it achieves its goals at its own speed and in its own way, and we accept the journey, allowing the water to flow consistently, doing what it needs to do to mould us into what we're becoming a tiny bit more each day.

There are several ways in which we can try too hard

Firstly, we might read about the experiences of other people when they do Reiki, when they self-treat, when they treat other people, when they receive attunements or empowerments. These people might experience particular things, see colours, have a particular sensation or a strong reaction and we might not be experiencing these things at the moment.

We think to ourselves, "I'm not doing it properly, I need to focus more, I need to do this better, I need to try harder to get it just right".

Well, no you don't.

We all have our own individual experiences when using Reiki. There are some people who see colours who wish they could feel tingling in their hands more. There are people whose hands fizz like crazy who wish they could see colours, and there are people who have very few sensations or experiences who wish they could experience something more than they currently are.

And things aren't set in stone, so what we experience now when using Reiki isn't representative of what we will notice as the energy flows. Things change, and we can develop our sensitivity to the energy through practice and through using special meditations that I have on my web site.

But what is not going to help is trying really hard, because Reiki works best, Reiki flows best when the person channelling the energy is chilled out and laid-back, just gently there with the energy, letting it happen, whatever is happening.

Just let it happen

Trying hard is a good way to put up barriers and slow your progress: they best way to progress with your Reiki is basically to give up and stop trying to do anything… just be there with the energy, no expectations, neutral, empty.

Just be, be mindful, notice what there is to notice, and if nothing's there to notice then notice that!

You will progress fastest when you stand aside metaphorically, do the exercises, just follow the instructions, be unconcerned by what you feel or don't feel, treat people, go through the motions, be unconcerned with what colours you might or might not see – it doesn't matter: be empty and compassionate and that's it.

Intuitive working

Another area where Reiki people might try too hard is when learning to work intuitively, and at Reiki Evolution we teach our students a method where they learn to allow their hands to drift with the energy to the right places to treat.

This approach works well for most people, though there are some whose intuition comes to them more in terms of images or words or an inner knowing, and that's fine too. But our basic approach is through hands drifting with the energy, rather like the hands being drawn like magnets to the right areas to treat, different from one person to another and from one session to another with the same person.

The key to success with our intuitive method is to not try: trying is actually the best way to stop it working, and the challenge that our students face is to learn to not do anything and not force anything, just to let it happen.

I remember a course that I ran in Cumbria several years ago where I was teaching this intuitive approach to Reiki practitioners and Masters. There were about 15-20 people on the course, we had treatment tables set up and there were perhaps 3-4 people to each table. One person was on the treatment couch and the others stood around the table practising allowing the energy to guide their hands. They all took turns on the table so everyone had the chance to practise on a few different people.

The method seemed to be working well for everyone except one poor girl whose hands were motionless, and remained motionless no matter how hard she tried to make the technique work. Of course it was her attempts to force it which were preventing her from achieving success with this method.

So what I did was to come and stand behind her and rest my hands on her shoulders.

Within a minute her hands started to drift. Now, this is not because I was giving her some sort of an 'energy boost' but because she was starting to have a bit of a Reiki treatment, and you know the feeling of melting and drifting and relaxing that this can bring, just within seconds. After a few moments she didn't care what was happening with her hands, she gave up trying, she drifted with the treatment – the merged with the energy – and her hands began to move to the right places to treat.

Having proved to herself that she could actually do this, she then went on to make the method work for her several times;

she made it work by not trying to make it work, by giving up and not trying, by just being, in neutral, merged and empty.

And that's a good approach for Reiki work in general, I think.

(7) You don't need to be perfect

Along with the need to be relaxed and laid-back and light-hearted about your Reiki practice, certainly not trying too hard, you should also make sure you're not beating yourself up for not being perfect.

Now, there is a precept that deals with this: just for today I will be compassionate towards myself and others, and that means forgiveness amongst other things: forgiveness for others and forgiveness for yourself.

Believing that you need to be perfect in everything that you do is an insidious belief and something that should not apply to your practice of Reiki. Just to make this completely clear: you do not need to be perfect to obtain benefits for yourself through Reiki, you do not need to be perfect when you're treating other people for them to receive all the benefits of Reiki.

Many different approaches work with Reiki, there is no exact way that things have to be done or carried out before they'll work, and Reiki is very accommodating.

But my mind wanders

Perhaps you mind wanders when you're treating someone.

So what?

This happens to everyone else and it'll happen to you. You will not mess up a Reiki treatment or be ineffective as a channel just because you were thinking about shopping for a while when you treated someone.

But how do you deal with a wandering mind?

Well, what you don't do is to try and force yourself to have an 'empty mind' – that will not work at all; that will make things worse because you now have two lots of thoughts: the original thoughts and all the new thoughts about getting rid of the first lot of thoughts!

Don't worry. Pay the thoughts no attention.

No need to focus on them. Just let them pass.

It doesn't matter, just bring your attention gently back to what you were doing, being mindful, merging with the energy and the recipient, letting it happen. And that's all you need to do, just be gentle with yourself.

Be light-hearted and compassionate

Will your mind wander again, having done that?

Probably, so just go through the procedure again: be light-hearted about it, be compassionate, let the thoughts go and bring your attention back to what you were doing.

Some treatments will probably be better than others in terms of a wandering mind, it'll sort itself out over time, and your mind will probably always wander some of the time. It doesn't matter. Do your best, make sure you're not forcing anything, and don't worry about it.

You're allowed to be human!

And there are other areas where you may well not do things perfectly, exactly according to the instructions, and it doesn't matter. If you're doing a self-treatment and you get the order of the hand positions wrong, it doesn't matter: Reiki will still flow, you'll still receive the benefit of the energy.

Maybe you realise that you forgot a stage that you usually carry out when treating someone: have you messed it up so they won't receive any benefit? No, Reiki will still have given them what they need.

Reiki is simple, Reiki works simply, Reiki rises above any set of rituals and rules that we might choose to follow, or forget to follow. You have a healing intent, and Reiki will follow that, and that is sufficient, no matter what you might say to yourself, or forget to say, or forget to do.

So don't worry.

Errors in Reiki attunements

Perhaps you're carrying out a Reiki attunement and you realise that you've missed out a section. Do you need to go back and do it all over again, apologising to the student for mis-attuning them?

No, it will still have worked fine.

There are so many different attunement styles in existence, with many different conflicting stages. Some attunements use a particular ritual that isn't present in other systems, other systems use stages that aren't present in your system. What is most important about attuning someone is your underlying intent, and the exact details of the ritual that you are using aren't so important.

By all means do your very best to carry out your attunement ritual according to the instructions that you were given, but also realise that there are no vital stages other than setting a definite intent when you begin; the rest is the icing on the cake, a set of movements, different in different lineages, that just help to remind you of what you want to happen, to support or focus your intent.

So you're fine.

You can be human.

(8) Don't keep trying to puzzle out 'why'

We've seen that the best state of mind to have when treating someone is to be empty and neutral, merged with the energy and merged with the recipient. We are in a mindful state, just being, not forcing things, letting it happen. If our mind wanders then we just gently bring our attention back to what we were doing, and bliss out on the energy.

And it would be nice if we could bring that lovely, centred, unconcerned state into other areas of our life, too, particularly when it comes to seeking answers or explanations for everything that is happening to us and to the people that we are treating.

Because if we seek answers or explanations for every little sensation that we have, every little happening, and particularly if we can't be content with a practice or an approach without understanding exactly why we are doing a particular thing, then we are going to make our journey with Reiki a particularly difficult one.

What do colours mean?

If you see a particular colour, or colours, when treating someone, or when self-treating, it might be nice just to accept this as a pretty light-show, an added bonus, a colourful and welcome side-effect of the flow of energy... rather than trying to puzzle out why you had a particular colour and what that means.

Maybe the colour does have a meaning – there are colours associated with the chakras for example – and maybe the energy was focusing on a particular chakra when you saw that colour. But because Reiki works on so many levels, because it deals with physical things, mental states, emotions, spiritual aspects, because it deals with historical problems that are still present in some way in our energy body, and it deals with things that are 'on the boil' and haven't manifested yet… we have no real idea of what it's doing other than to be safe in the knowledge that the energy is giving us or the recipient what we need.

So stop trying to puzzle things out: it will make no difference to your experience of the energy or the effectiveness of your Reiki.

Get your head out of the equation and just let the energy do what it needs to do, without all that frantic mental activity!

What do sensations mean?

If you have a particular sensation when treating someone, or you were drawn to a particular area of the body, do you really need to know why that happened?

If your hands ends up resting on someone's liver area, does that mean they have liver disease?

No, it doesn't, it just means that the energy needs to flow there to produce the balance that is appropriate for the recipient.

We don't diagnose with Reiki: Doctors diagnose. Reiki Practitioners and Reiki Masters don't diagnose, and shouldn't diagnose, and if they feel an urge to diagnose something then they should stop it.

In any case, Reiki works on lots of levels, so in Traditional Chinese Medicine the liver is said to hold mental states and emotions that might be being dealt with; is that what's happening? Who knows? We don't need to know, we can just accept that Reiki is doing what it needs to do, and go with the flow, merging with the energy in a lovely mindful state.

Let's speculate!

Worse still is the urge to try and come up with our own theories about what we are feeling.

Some people start to think in terms of blockages or negative energy or, worse still, 'dark energy'. Those are not helpful terms to use when talking to a Reiki client, who came in looking forward to a lovely blissful session and come out with a belief that they are harbouring a blockage or dark energy.

We don't need to introduce such ideas into our Reiki because they're not helpful to us or the people that we work on.

The sooner we can accept that Reiki is all a bit mysterious and puzzling, but works tremendously well, so we can just let it do what it needs to do without second guessing what's happening, the better it will be for us because we can just let go of all those questions and enjoy the journey.

Did I really feel that?

Actually, along with thinking too much and questioning everything comes the challenge that we can face when second-guessing things that we feel or notice.

Did I really feel that sensation, was I making it up, is it all in my head, did I only feel something because I wanted to?

Well, either you feel something or you don't. If you feel something you can trust that you felt it; you can't make yourself feel something. If it was possible to fool yourself into feeling Reiki sensations then everyone would feel something and there would be no-one who was concerned that they don't feel anything when doing Reiki... they would all have magicked sensations into existence, wouldn't they?

So just accept and go with what you feel: if you notice a lot of energy flowing into a part of someone's body (maybe your hands are fizzing or tingling or pulsing or whatever sensation you have) then just stay there for longer until you feel the flow of energy subside.

You can trust what you're feeling.

You're not making it up.

(9) Trust your intuition

Along with doubts about whether people are fooling themselves when they notice the flow of energy, come doubts about a person's intuitive ability.

Am I really feeling drawn to that part of the body or am I fooling myself? I heard a word or phrase in my head, or I saw an image, is this all in my head? Am I making it up?

Did my hand really feel like it was being pulled like a magnet to the person's knee, or is this only because I know that they had an injury there?

You need to know something: you are intuitive. Everyone is intuitive.

You may not be used to noticing the intuitive messages that your body and mind are sending you, but they have always been there.

Are you making it up? Yes, in a way: nobody else is giving you this information, it's coming from you, from that intuitive part of you that generates such messages and insights, or that 'inner knowing'.

Intuition can come to you in different ways

Maybe when treating someone you feel strangely drawn to a particular area of their body, your attention wants to rest there or dwell there. It might not make any sense, but that doesn't matter.

Just go with what's coming to you and direct the energy there, resting your hands or hovering your hands over that area.

Maybe when you're self-treating, you feel drawn to a particular area of your body, well just focus your attention there and allow the energy to flow there.

Just accept what comes to you and work with it.

Some people have intuition come to them in terms of visual images or words or muscle movements: everyone's different. Don't assume that this isn't real intuition, that because it's you and you're not intuitive, this can only be just nonsense.

Just stop thinking and stop worrying and stop second-guessing yourself, and cultivate the lovely mindful state that you enjoy when giving Reiki.

Ease into that lovely merged state and just accept what's coming to you, allowing the energy to guide you in its own way, because you are already as intuitive as you need to be, and the way to access your intuition is to just merge with the energy, and let it happen.

(10) Ignore silly rules and restrictions

Another problem with thinking too much is that we can start to overcomplicate something that is a very simple and a very safe way of helping ourselves and helping other people to change things for the better. And if we think too much, and particularly if we start to worry too much – and I have to say that there is something in the Reiki precepts about worry – we end up with people speculating about potential dangers, imaginary dangers, problems that have no basis in anyone's experience, and we start to limit our practice of Reiki.

And you can see that in different lineages, where students are taught long lists of situations where they shouldn't use Reiki, people that they shouldn't treat, things that they have to do, or should always do, or should never do, and many of these restrictions and limitations are just complete nonsense, completely divorced from reality.

And students take these teaching on in good faith, and pass them on to their students when they become teachers, never questioning whether what they were taught has any basis in fact or experience.

Reiki contraindications

So what restrictions do we have careering around the world of Reiki? Take a look at these examples:

- You shouldn't treat people who are wearing contact lenses

- You shouldn't treat people who have cancer
- You shouldn't treat babies
- You shouldn't treat people who have a broken bone
- You shouldn't treat pregnant women
- You shouldn't treat people with high blood pressure
- You shouldn't treat people who have pacemakers
- You shouldn't treat diabetics
- You shouldn't treat people who are stressed.

These are nonsense and have no basis because Reiki is a safe and nurturing energy that gives people what they need.

So, where is the evidence that using Reiki makes people's pacemakers explode? Where is the research paper that proves this? Or even if there isn't a research paper, where are the anecdotes, where it is clear that Reiki messed up a pacemaker?

Where is the evidence? There is none.

Where is the evidence that you shouldn't treat people who are stressed? There is none.

Good grief this is nonsense isn't it?

Some people are taught that you shouldn't treat clients with cancer because the Reiki will 'feed the cancer'. OK, where's the evidence? And also, since everyone listening to this track has some cancer cells in their body, cells that have gone wrong and which are mopped up routinely by our immune system, we shouldn't be treating anyone, including ourselves!

It would be a death sentence.

Some people are taught that they shouldn't treat pregnant women. OK, where's the evidence that Reiki is dangerous? There is none, of course. But because sometimes women can be pregnant without knowing it yet, particularly in the early stages, if you believe that Reiki is dangerous to pregnant women then you should be refusing to treat any woman of childbearing age just to make sure that you're not treating someone who might be pregnant.

And if you're attuned to Reiki yourself, then of course you would need to make sure that you never had children.

It's all about worrying too much

What all these rules and restrictions do is to introduce into Reiki something that Reiki is designed to ease: worry, worry about what's going to happen, restricting what we do 'just to be on the safe side', all based on wild and feverish imaginings that are passed on from teacher to student.

Well, Reiki is bigger than that and need not be restricted.

And another area where Reiki does not need to be restricted is in terms of what we are told that we have to do in order to work with Reiki.

There are Reiki people out there who have been taught a fifteen-stage process or ritual that they need to go through before they start a Reiki treatment. If they don't get it right, well they've been told that it isn't going to work properly and so they worry about that, as you would, but of course such rituals are optional: you don't have to go through a 15-stage process before you give someone a Reiki treatment.

Someone somewhere made up the ritual and then it's ended up being passed on to people as gospel, as dogma.

There are some Reiki people out there who have been taught that they have to draw the Reiki symbols on their palms every day because if they don't then the symbols won't work for them. People are told that you have to draw the three Reiki symbols over your palms before you give someone a treatment, or that you have to draw the three symbols over every hand position that you use.

Reiki is very simple, you know

You plonk your hands on someone, shut your eyes if you like, and the energy flows.

Much more than that is really gilding the lily.

And I know that some rituals can be useful: they help you to focus your attention, they help you to focus your intent in a particular way, and some people like rituals and there's nothing wrong with that.

But we should remember that Reiki is a very simple system, it works brilliantly without clutter, and if we use processes and visualisations and set phrases, we should remember that these are actually optional, not compulsory.

We can experiment and find our own comfortable way with the energy, different from the way that other people work, and that's fine.

The Ten Rules of Reiki in a few sentences

If I was going to try and sum up the ten rules of Reiki in just a few sentences, I would say this:

To get the most out of your Reiki, I recommend that you make a commitment to yourself to work on yourself daily in some way as your top priority, but not beating yourself up if you miss the occasional day.

Use energy exercises, self-treat, focus on the precepts regularly and drip-feed mindfulness into your daily activities and routines.

Don't try too hard, though: be light-hearted and forgiving towards yourself because you don't have to be perfect.

Try not to clutter your mind with lots of thoughts and doubts and questions: just be neutral, have no expectations, be empty and content.

And make sure you keep things simple. Reiki works best when it's simple.

Fundamentals

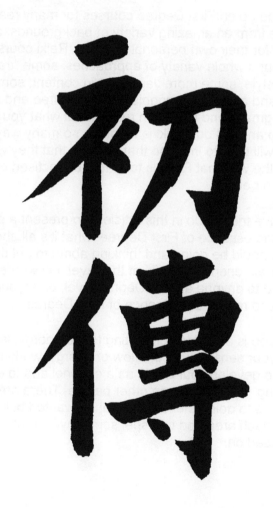

Back to Basics: Reiki First Degree

People end up on First Degree courses for many reasons and come from an amazing variety of backgrounds, all attending for their own personal reasons. Reiki courses in the UK present a whole variety of approaches, some "traditional" Western-style, some more Japanese in content, some wildly different and almost unrecognisable, some free and intuitive, others dogmatic and based on rules about what you should always do and not do. Reiki is taught in so many ways, and students will tend to imagine that the way that they were taught is the way that Reiki is taught and practised by most other Reiki people.

What I have tried to do in this article is to present a simple guide to the essence of First Degree: what it's all about and what we should be doing and thinking about to get the most out of our experience of Reiki at this level. My words are addressed to anyone at First Degree level, or anyone who would like to review the essence of First Degree.

First Degree is all about connecting to the energy, learning to develop your sensitivity to the flow of energy, working on yourself to develop your ability as a channel and to enhance self-healing, and working on other people. There are many approaches to doing these things, and I wanted below to touch on each area and to dispel some myths that may have been passed on.

Connecting to the energy

On your Reiki course you will have received some attunements or some empowerments. Attunements are not standard rituals within the world of Reiki and take many forms, some simpler and some more complex. They have evolved and changed greatly during their journey from teacher to teacher in the West. There is no "right way" to carry out an attunement and the individual details of a ritual do not matter a great deal. They all work.

Equally, there is no "correct" number of attunements that have to be carried out at First Degree level. The number four is quoted often as being the "correct" number but this has no basis in Reiki's original form, and whether you receive one, two, three or four rituals on your course, that is fine.

On your course you may have received some "empowerments" rather than attunements, though these are less common. The word "empowerment", or "Reiju empowerment", refers to a connection ritual that has come to us from some Japanese sources, and is closer in essence to the empowerment that Mikao Usui conveyed to his students. Again, there is no correct number of empowerments that has to be carried out. One is enough but it is nice to do more.

What we experience when receiving an attunement or an empowerment will vary a lot. Some people have fireworks and bells and whistles and that's nice for them; other people notice a lot less, very little, or even nothing, and that's fine too. What we feel when we have an attunement is not a guide to how well it has worked for us. Attunements work, and sometimes we will have a strong experience, but it's not compulsory! Whether we have noticed a lot, or very little, the attunement will have given us what we need.

Since in Mikao Usui's system you would have received empowerments from him again and again, it would be nice if you could echo this practice by receiving further empowerments (or attunements) and perhaps these might be available at your teacher's Reiki shares or get-togethers, if they hold them. But it is possible to receive distant Reiju empowerments and various teachers make them freely available as a regular 'broadcast'. This is not essential, and your connection to Reiki once given does not fizzle out, but it would be a beneficial practice if you could receive regular empowerments from someone.

Developing your Sensitivity to the energy

People's experience of energy when they first start working with Reiki can vary. Some people notice more than others, particularly in the early stages, and if we perhaps notice less going on in our hands when compared with another student on the course we can become disillusioned to an extent: that little voice in your head says "I know Reiki works for everyone... but it's not going to work for me. I knew it wasn't going to work for me". Well if this describes your situation then I can say to you that Reiki will work for you, and is working for you, and the vast majority of Reiki people can feel the flow of energy through them in some way, though your particular 'style' of sensing the energy may not involve the more usual heat, fizzing, tingling, pulsing etc. that many people experience.

There are a few Reiki Master/Teachers out there who feel absolutely nothing in their hands, but this is not common, and Reiki is still working for them.

Sensitivity to the flow of energy develops over time, with practice. Some people are lucky enough to be able to feel quite a lot in their hands and in their bodies to begin with, but others have to be patient, trust that Reiki is working for them, and perhaps focus more on the feedback that they receive from the people that they treat, rather than what they feel – or don't feel – in their hands.

It would be worthwhile if all First Degree students spent some time regularly practising feeling energy: between your hands, around your cat or dog or your pot plant or a tree, around someone else's head and shoulders, over someone's supine body, noticing any differences in the sensation in your hands as you move your hands from one place to another.

Don't expect to experience a particular thing or a particular intensity of feeling. Be neutral and simply notice what experience you have and how that experience might change from one area to another.

On some First Degree courses this process will be taught as "scanning", where you hover your hands over the recipient's body, drift your hands from one place to another, and notice any areas which are drawing more energy. This can provide some useful information in terms of suggesting additional or alternative hand-positions to use when you treat, and can suggest areas where you are going to spend longer when you treat.

Working on yourself

It is vital that after going on a First Degree course you establish a regular routine of working on yourself in order to develop your fledgling ability as a channel and to obtain the benefits that Reiki can provide in terms of balancing your life and self-healing. Most people decide to learn Reiki because they are looking for some personal benefits as well as looking to help other people, and the way to get the most out of the Reiki system is to work on yourself regularly.

On your First Degree course you will have been taught a self-treatment method, perhaps a Japanese-style meditation but more likely the Western "hands-on" self-treatment method. You will most likely have been given a set of hand-positions to use, but please remember that these positions are not set in stone and, particularly if some of the hand positions are quite uncomfortable to use in practice, you will develop your own style.

It is fine to change the hand positions based on what feels right from one self-treatment to another, and you should do what feels appropriate. There is no "correct" set of positions that you have to use, and each hand-position does not have to be held for a particular period of time. Treat for however long you have time for, and however long feels right for each hand-position you decide to use.

Many people are taught that they have to do a "21 day self-treat", and some people have the impression that they then do not need to self-treat any more. The "21 day" period has no real basis, and I can say that you ought to be thinking in terms of working on yourself long-term. To gain the greatest benefits from this wonderful system you need to persevere and make working with energy a permanent feature of your life with Reiki, a basic background practice, the effects of which will build up cumulatively as you continue to work with the energy.

You may have been taught a series of energy exercises and meditations called "Hatsurei ho" which comes from Japanese Reiki, and I can commend this practice to you. It is a wonderful way of grounding, balancing, and enhancing you ability as a channel, and should be a regular part of your Reiki routine.

Treating other people

First Degree is also about starting to work on other people, a process which also benefits the giver, so plus points all round really! A few students may have been taught not to treat others at First Degree, or for a particular prescribed period, but this is an unnecessary restriction and Reiki can be shared with other people straight away.

There are many different approaches to treating others, and we should not get bogged down with too many rules and regulations about how we 'must' proceed. Reiki can be approached in quite a regimented way in some lineages, and students may worry that if they are not remembering all the stages that they 'have' to carry out then they will not be carrying out the treatment properly. This is an unnecessary worry because treating other people is simple.

So here is a simple approach that you can use: close your eyes, maybe put your hands in the prayer position, and take a few long deep breaths to calm you and still your mind. You should have in mind that the energy you will channel should be for the highest good of the recipient, but there is no particular form of words that you need to use when commencing your treatment.

Now we are going to focus your attention on connecting to the energy. Imagine that energy is flooding down to you from above, flooding through your crown, through the centre of your body, down to your Dantien (an energy centre two fingerbreadths below your tummy button and 1/3rd of the way into your body). Imagine the energy building up and intensifying there. You are filling with energy.

Now direct your attention towards the recipient and imagine that you are merging with them, becoming one with them. Feel compassion and enjoy the moment.

You may now begin your treatment, and maybe it would be nice to rest your hands on their shoulders for a while, to connect to them and to get the energy flowing. What hand positions you use will vary depending on what you were taught – there are many variations – and they are all variations on a theme, a way of firing the energy from lots of different directions to give it the best chance of getting to where it needs to go.

Hand-positions for treating others are not set in stone and do not have to be followed slavishly.

They are just there as a set of guidelines to follow to build your confidence when treating others, and with time and practice you will start to leave behind these basic instructions and gear any treatment towards the needs of the recipient on that occasion, perhaps based on what you picked up when you were 'scanning' and perhaps based on intuitive impressions, where you feel drawn to a particular area of the body.

Don't try and work out 'why' you have felt drawn to a particular area of the body: just accept your impression and go with it.

Reiki is basically a hands-on treatment method, though for reasons of comfort and propriety you will choose to hover your hands over the recipient in some areas rather than resting on the body. I do not plaster my hands over the recipient's face or throat, for example, because I think that this is uncomfortable and unsettling for the person you are working on.

You do not have to hover your hands for every hand position, as some people are taught, and equally you do not have to keep at least one hand in physical contact with the recipient's body at all times, for fear of 'losing' your connection: your connection to the recipient is a state of mind, and where your hands are is irrelevant!

As you treat, you should aim to feel yourself merging with the energy, becoming one with the energy, to imagine yourself disappearing into the energy, and this can give you a quite blissful experience. Your mind may wander, particularly in the early stages of your Reiki practice, but you do not need to worry about this.

If you notice thoughts intruding, pay them no attention; let them drift on like clouds.

If you make a big effort to try and get rid of your thoughts then you will have in your head the original thoughts and then all the new thoughts about getting rid of the first lot of thoughts… you have made things worse! Just bring your attention gently back to the recipient, to the energy, feel yourself disappearing into the energy, merging with the recipient, and let the energy flow; your treatment can become a wonderful meditation.

It is not acceptable to chat to other people while giving a Reiki treatment.

If you want to be an effective channel for the energy then you need to direct your attention to the work at hand and make sure you are not unduly distracted. For this reason, conversation between yourself and the recipient should be restricted. Reiki works best of you are still and focused, merging with the energy, in a gentle meditative state. Developing this state takes practice and you can't do it properly if you are chatting.

You do not need to stay for a particular set amount of time for each hand position.

Though it would be probably be best to stay for a few minutes in each position, if in a particular hand position you feel a lot of energy coming through your hands then you can stay in that position for longer – sometimes a lot longer – until the sensation subsides and you can then move onto the next area. Your hands can guide you.

Work from the head and shoulders, down the length of the body, and it is nice to finish with the ankles.

Many people are taught to smooth down the energy field at the end of a session, and that is a nice thing to do, but remember that you do not have to follow any rituals slavishly, particularly in terms of any sort of 'closing' ritual; you do not need to touch the ground, you do not need to say a particular set of words, you do not need to visualise anything in particular, and you do not need to make any 'set' movements of your hands or body.

The Reiki Precepts

On your First Degree course you will have been introduced to the Reiki Precepts, or Reiki Principles, Mikao Usui's "rules to live by'". Just in case you have been given a slightly distorted version of the precepts, here is a more accurate translation:

> *The secret of inviting happiness through many blessings*
> *The spiritual medicine for all illness*
>
> *For today only: Do not anger; Do not worry*
> *Be humble*
> *Be honest in your dealings with people*
> *Be compassionate to yourself and others*
>
> *Do gassho every morning and evening*
>
> *Keep in your mind and recite*
>
> *The founder, Usui Mikao*

Any reference to 'honouring your elders, parents and teachers' is a later addition to the list, and is not what Mikao Usui taught.

The precepts were the hub of the whole system, and it is said that as much spiritual development can come through following the precepts in your daily life as would come from any energy work, so they are important.

If we can try to focus on living in the moment, not forever dwelling on the past or worrying about the future (fear is a distraction), if we can remind ourselves of the many blessings we have in our lives, if we can forgive ourselves for not being perfect and if we can see things from another's point of view, if we can be compassionate towards ourselves as well as others, then we have gone a long way towards achieving a liberating sense of serenity and contentment. This is not something to be achieved overnight, of course: it is a work-in-progress.

Finally

Reiki has the potential to make an amazing, positive difference to you and the people around you. Remember that Reiki is simplicity itself, and by taking some steps to work on yourself regularly, and share Reiki with the people close to you, you are embarking on a very special journey.

How far you travel on that journey is governed by how many steps you take.

The Precepts

Mikao Usui gave his students a series of 'precepts' to follow. The Concise Oxford Dictionary (9th Edition) defines a precept as (1) a command, a rule of conduct, and (2) a moral instruction, and they are an important part of Buddhist practice.

We know that Mikao Usui was a Tendai Buddhist, and so precepts would have been an important part of his spiritual life. Lay followers of Buddhism generally undertake to follow (at least one of) five precepts, which are given in the form of promises to oneself: "I will (try) to...". Here are the five Buddhist precepts:

1. To refrain from harming living creatures (killing).
2. To refrain from taking that which is not freely given (stealing).
3. To refrain from sexual misconduct.
4. To refrain from incorrect speech (lying, harsh language, slander, idle chit-chat).
5. To refrain from intoxicants which lead to loss of mindfulness.

So precepts are a list of guidelines for living your life. They are not framed in terms of "thou shalt not..." as in the Judaeo-Christian tradition but rather are a set of ideals to work towards, recommendations about thought and behaviour that you should follow as much as you can.

Everyone who has learned Reiki will have, or should have, seen the Reiki precepts – Mikao Usui's 'rules to live by' – and they are available in a variety of different forms in different lineages.

Usui's precepts aren't what is commonly taught in the West

There is actually some difference between the precepts that Mikao Usui was teaching and the precepts that are quoted commonly in the West. For example, some Western versions of the precepts include an extra item: "honour your parents, elders and teachers". This is not original and seems to have been added by Mrs Takata to make the "list of rules to live by" more acceptable to her (largely) Christian American audience.

There has been some speculation about where Mikao Usui's precepts come from. It has been claimed that they originate in a book that was published in Usui's time, and it has been claimed that they are based on the edicts of Mutsuhito, the Meiji Emperor.

Certainly it seems that many Tendai and Zen Buddhist teachers were passing on similar principles in Usui Sensei's time.

But now we know that Usui's precepts were his wording of an earlier set of precepts that have been traced back to the early 9th century, precepts that were used in a Tendai sect of Shugendo with which Usui Sensei was in contact.

These precepts were a way of addressing aspects of the Buddhist eight-fold path in a simplified form, and they are the very 'hub' of the whole system.

The precepts were the baseline, the foundation of Usui Sensei's teachings, and it was thought that individual could achieve as much spiritual development by following the precepts as could be achieved by carrying out all the energy exercises.

Aren't negative affirmations a bad idea?

Incidentally, you may find some commentators saying that negative affirmations are not a good idea: such things are said to be more effective when framed in positive terms.

What we have presented to us in the precepts is just a quirk of translation from Japanese to English: the precepts are actually a recommendation that we exist in the moment in a state where we are free from anger and worry, a 'worry-free, anger-free' state.

For me, Mikao Usui's precepts represent both some of the beneficial effects that Reiki can produce in your life if you work with the energy regularly, and they represent a set of principles that we need to follow to enhance our journey of self-healing and self-development with Reiki.

My main purpose in writing this article is to introduce you to a way of working with the precepts in conjunction with the Reiki energy. This is something that I have been experimenting with: a way of directly experiencing the effects of a precept in terms of energy flow.

I would like to suggest that you do the following, for a couple of minutes at a time, twice a day, for a month: Sit with your eyes closed and your hands resting in your lap, palms up. You are going to be releasing energy through your hands.

Stage One

Sit comfortably with your eyes closed and your hands resting in your lap, palms up. Take a few long deep breaths and feel yourself becoming peaceful and relaxed. Your mind empties. Say to yourself "I now release all my anger..."; say this three times to yourself if you like. Allow energy to be released through your palms, and be still until the flow of energy subsides. This may take a little while, particularly the first time you try this exercise.

Stage Two

Now say to yourself "I now release all my worry..."; say this three times to yourself if you like. Again allow a flurry of energy to leave your hands and be still until it subsides. Again this may take a little while, particularly the first time you try this exercise.

Alternatively, try carrying out the releasing exercise in time with your breath. Breathe in gently, say to yourself "I now release all my anger..." and then breathe out, allowing your anger to flood out of you on the out breath. Gently breath in, and repeat.

Mindfulness and Compassion

In this article I want to talk about Mindfulness and Compassion, which I believe are two essential components of Reiki practice. Whether we are treating others, working on ourselves, empowering others or living our lives with Reiki, we should grow to embody those two states, the essence of the Reiki precepts.

Mindfulness

According to Usui Sensei's surviving students, Mikao Usui introduced his students to the practice of mindfulness at First Degree level, and emphasised this more at Second Degree level. According to the Concise Oxford Dictionary (9th Edition), to be mindful is to take heed or care, to be conscious.

Mindfulness or being mindful is being aware of your present moment. You are not judging, reflecting or thinking. You are simply observing the moment in which you find yourself, fully aware. Moments are like a breath. Each breath is replaced by the next breath. You are there with no other purpose than being awake and aware of that moment.

So mindfulness is a state of living in the moment, of being relaxed, calm and fully engaged in what we are doing. Mindfulness is being fully aware of what is happening right now and giving ourselves completely to our task without distraction. By learning how to enjoy and be in the present moment we can find peace within ourselves.

Like precepts, mindfulness is largely associated with Buddhism and it is a meditative practice that is not reserved for special meditation sessions: it is a practice that you can embrace as part of your daily life and when carrying out routine and mundane tasks.

The best guide that I have found to the use of mindfulness as part of your daily life is the following book, written by Thich Nhat Hanh: "The Miracle of Mindfulness" and I recommend that all Reiki practitioners and teachers obtain a copy and practise being mindful during their daily activities.

I believe that Mikao Usui's precepts are all about mindfulness, and that when we are exhorted by the precepts to "just for today" release anger and worry, we are being guided to exist as far as we can in a mindful state.

Anger and worry are distractions, you see, and if we can exist in the moment by being mindful then we will not dwell on the past and beat ourselves up for things that did not go the way we wanted, and we will not dwell on the future, perhaps worrying about things that have not yet happened.

We can learn to release our attachments to the past and the future and just "be" now, content and accepting in the moment, by learning to be mindful.

Compassion

The final precept, that of being "compassionate towards ourselves and others" is for me an exhortation to be gentle with ourselves, to be patient, to be light-hearted, to not take ourselves quite so seriously and above all to be forgiving – first of all of ourselves but also of others. By accepting and forgiving ourselves we start to release our anger and our worry, and move towards a state of contentment in the moment.

The original system was a spiritual path, a path to enlightenment, and the precepts were what Usui Sensei's system was all about. These principles are a foundation for everything we do with Reiki: the states of mindfulness and compassion arise from following the precepts and from working with Reiki.

For example, how do we feel when we carry out a Reiki treatment? Treating someone with Reiki is a special, special gift. We feel a closeness, an intimacy, a merging with the recipient; we receive trust and we experience compassion. Ideally we should just be there in the moment, with the energy, with the recipient, with no expectations.

We do not treat someone with the intention to resolve their health problem or eliminate their headache. We just merge with the energy and allow Reiki to do its work; we create a sacred space for healing to occur. If our mind wanders, as it may do, then we notice this and gently but firmly bring our attention back to the present and what we are doing. We become one with the energy as it flows through us, we become one with the recipient, and we experience that blissful contentment in the moment.

When we treat we are mindful: we are an observer, not a participant.

Though some are taught that you can hold a conversation with someone as you treat, or watch television at the same time, this really will not lead to the best being given to the recipient. To be the most effective channel we can be, we need to be there with the energy, fully and gently engaged in our work, giving ourselves fully to the task without distraction.

Those same principles apply when working on ourselves, whether carrying out Hatsurei ho or self-treating. The state we should seek to achieve is that of being fully engaged in the endeavour, of being with the energy without distraction, merged, aware and simply existing in the moment, with a gentle feeling of forgiveness, love and compassion towards ourselves.

So both Mindfulness and Compassion are fundamental to our life with Reiki, fundamental to the Reiki precepts, to working on others and working on ourselves.

Not surprisingly they are also an essential component of the transmission of Reiki to another person through carrying out Reiju empowerments. Reiju is the 'connection ritual' that Usui Sensei used, and taught to his surviving students. It is simple, elegant and powerful, free from the clutter and detail that surrounds most Western attunement styles.

When we perform Reiju we have no expectations: we are there in the moment with the energy, following the prescribed movements. We are relaxed and fully engaged in what we are doing, aware of what is happening right now, and we give ourselves completely to our task without distraction. That is the essence of Reiju, the essence of treatments, the essence of the precepts, and the essence of our life with Reiki.

How to start a Reiki treatment

A simple ritual to get your Reiki treatment started

People in different lineages are taught different ways of starting off a Reiki treatment – the ritual(s) that you carry out to get things started – and I thought it would be useful to share with you the sequence that we teach on Reiki Evolution courses, so that you can compare it with what you were taught.

It might trigger off some ideas and help you to develop your own way of doing things if you wanted to.

When standing by the recipient, our students are taught to go through a sequence represented by the letters A, C, B, M, F.

A = Affirm
C = Connect
B = Build
M = Merge
F = Flow

Below I describe these stages in a bit more detail…

Affirm

It's quite common, I think, for Reiki people to make some sort of affirmation or dedication before starting a Reiki treatment, and we have students silently affirm, "I dedicate this treatment to the highest good of [client's name]".

It's just a nice way of reminding yourself that when you carry out a Reiki treatment, you do so in a 'neutral' way, with no expectation of a particular result, metaphorically standing aside to allow the energy to be drawn by the recipient to where it needs to go. So you're setting the right intent.

Once you have gone through this process again and again with different clients, you probably don't need to keep on reminding and re-reminding yourself at the start of each session: you know what your intent is.

Connect

Here is where we focus our attention on our 'connection' to the energy, and we have our students imagine that energy is flowing down through their crown, down through the centre of the body to the Tanden.

And just focusing on that for a little while can bring a lovely meditative state, ideal for carrying out a Reiki treatment on someone.

Build

Now we direct our attention towards the Tanden, that energy centre two finger-breadths below your tummy button and 1/3rd of the way into your body.

This is the centre of your personal universe, the location of your intuition and creativity, a part of the body that is focused on in many traditional practices, for example martial arts, flower arranging, even the tea ceremony.

Here we notice that the energy starts to build here, strengthening and intensifying.

Merge

Having focused on our 'connection' to the energy and the building up of Reiki within us, now we move our attention to the recipient on the treatment table before us, imagining that we are merging with them, becoming one with them, experiencing a state of oneness.

We are neutral, empty, with no expectations, a necessary bystander in the process that is to follow.

Flow

And finally, we allow the energy to flow, drawn by the recipient to the most appropriate places for them on that occasion.

We have established ourselves as a clear channel, a free-flowing conduit, stepping aside metaphorically to allow the energy to be drawn by the recipient, creating a 'healing space' that they can use for their highest good.

We follow the flow of energy, resting our hands in the areas that are drawing the most energy, staying there for as long as the energy needs to flow there, resting our hands in just the right places for that person on that occasion.

Though intuitive working is something that we focus on mainly on our Second Degree courses, some of our First Degree students find that they are already feeling guided by the energy and we encourage them to go with the flow, 'getting out of the way' – not worrying or trying to puzzle out why you are being drawn to a particular area, just letting it happen.

Nice and simple

So there is a simple sequence that you can follow.

I really like the way that it flows from a simple affirmation, noticing your connection to the energy and building the energy within you, moving your attention towards the recipient, merging with them and allowing the energy to flow.

It's like a lovely meditative dance with the energy.

Over to you

If this sequence differs from what you are doing currently, why not try it and see how you get on with it. And post a message below to let me know how it went.

Maybe there is something that you could incorporate into your own ritual, whatever that might be.

None of these things are set in stone, of course, and you can find your own distinctive way, so I hope the above has been helpful to you.

What hand positions should I use?

Are there hand positions that you should always use?

In some Reiki lineages, students are taught 'the' hand positions that they need to use, 'the' twelve hand positions, as if it were set in stone.

But do Reiki treatments really need to follow a set format, no matter what the energy needs of the client? Does every client have to be treated in exactly the same way?

I believe that having a set of hand positions to follow when you are starting out on your Reiki journey is very useful: you have some basic instructions to follow, you don't need to worry, and you can concentrate on getting used to working with the energy, becoming comfortable with being with people in a treatment setting.

You are firing the energy from lots of different directions to make sure it has the best chance to get to where it needs to.

But this 'one size fits all' approach is a bit limiting. Not everyone is the same, so why would we apply the same hand positions to everybody we treat?

So how might we start to adjust or alter where we are resting our hands?

Varying your hand positions for each client

There are two ways to adjust the hand positions that you use: through scanning and through intuition.

Scanning

"Scanning" is taught on most Reiki course and it is a way of finding out where the energy is flowing to on the client's body in the greatest amounts. Energy flowing strongly gives people a variety of sensations, and common feelings might be heat in your hands, or warmth, fizzing, tingling, buzzing, throbbing, heaviness, a magnetic feeling etc.

You hover your hands a few inches away from the client, drift your hand from one place to another, or sweep from one area to another, and focus your attention on the sensations that you are getting on your hand/fingers.

When doing this, you may notice that there are areas of need that don't tie in with the standard hand positions that you are taught, and you could add an extra hand position when you get that part of the body during your treatment, or alter the hand positions away from the standard ones, to accommodate this area of need.

Working intuitively

Intuition is another approach that can be used to gear your treatment more towards the energy needs of the person that you are working on.

Intuition can express itself in a person in different ways: a general 'impression', a feeling of being 'drawn' to an area of the body, an 'inner knowing', or you may find that your hands are drifting apparently of their own accord to some area. This latter approach is something that we teach on our Reiki courses, in the form of "Reiji ho", an intuitive approach that derives from Japanese Reiki.

So after starting off your treatment in whatever way you do that, you could then simply follow your impressions about where to rest your hands, and go with the flow.

How long should I spend in each hand position?

Treat like clockwork?

In some Reiki lineages, students are taught to spend a set amount of time treating each hand position, no matter who they are working on, and some practitioners use audio CDs with little 'bells' that sound out every three minutes, say.

But isn't this a bit mechanical, and everyone's different, so why would we give essentially the same treatment to everyone that we work on?

Altering your treatments to suit the client

The energy needs of each person that we work on will be different, so it's reasonable to expect each Reiki treatment that we give to be different, based on the individual energy needs of the client.

I don't think we should treat everyone like a "Reiki robot", changing hand position every time a bell pings, no matter what the client's energy system needs on that occasion. In my article "What hand positions should I use?" I spoke about moving beyond the standard hand positions that are taught in some lineages,and we can also move beyond the idea of treating for the same amount of time in each hand position.

Clients will have areas of the body that need Reiki more than others, so it makes sense to spend longer in these areas of need, and to spend less time in areas where there's not such a great need for Reiki to flow.

How to know how long to take in one position

So how can we work out how long we should spend in each hand position? I would like to suggest two methods, one based on sensing the flow of energy, and one based on intuition.

Most Reiki people can feel the flow of energy through their hands, which often shows itself as heat, fizzing, tingling, buzzing, heaviness, a magnetic feeling or whatever, if you can feel the flow of energy through your hands then you will be able to tell whether the hand position you are using is drawing lots of energy.

Sometimes it's completely clear, since your hands are absolutely 'on fire'!

It would be a good idea to stay in that hand position for longer, and after a while you will start to notice that the flow of energy – and associates sensations – starts to reduce in intensity.

When things have calmed down, move onto your next hand position.

We can also allow our intuition to guide us in terms of how long we spend working on a particular part of the body. Everyone is intuitive, and our intuition can make itself known to us in different ways. We may feel 'locked' into a particular hand position, or have an 'inner knowing' that we should stay where we are for the time being.

One little trick that I have used in the past to tell whether I need to stay where I am or move on involves using a visualisation that connects to your inner knowing: when treating someone, and I'm wondering whether I should move on now, I have an imaginary hand appear in my mind's eye, resting where my real hand is.

I imagine that this imaginary hand moves away from the body, as if on a piece of elastic, and if the imaginary hand wants to pull itself back to its original position, pulled by the elastic, then I should stay there for longer.

If the hand seems happy to drift away, in my mind's eye, then I know it's ok to move on to a new position… just a little visualisation that you can use to access intuitive knowledge.

Over to you

If these approaches are new to you, why not try them and see what happens, and let us know about your experiences by posting a message below.

Or maybe you started out doing treatments with standard timings, and now you don't.

How did that happen, and what do you think about the quality of your treatments now that you're working more freestyle?

Do I need to keep at least one hand on a person when I treat them?

Keep touching or you'll lose the 'connection'?

In some lineages, students are taught that they always need to keep at least one hand resting on the body at all times because, if they do not, they will 'lose their connection' with the client, and then have to go through a ritual again in order to regain that lost connection.

But is this really necessary?

Do we have to have to touch the body every second, like a sort of Reiki tag-team, for fear of disconnecting, and is the Reiki 'connection' so fragile?

What's the difference between hands-on and hands-off?

I believe that there is no difference between a Reiki treatment carried out when hands are resting on the body, and treatments where hands hover over the body.

Reiki is generally carried out as a 'hands-on' therapy and I think that this is a good idea: there is something very special and healing about human touch, with or without the addition of Reiki, and that closeness or connection that comes through making physical contact with another person is an important part of the Reiki experience.

Of course there are times – and hand positions – where it is better for the sake of propriety and respect to keep your hands off the body, particularly when working intuitively, when hands can end up wanting to go goodness-knows-where, and it's not always wise to always put your hands down where they want to come to rest!

Basically Reiki is a hands-on practice

Viewing Reiki as a hands-on practice, though, does not mean that we have to keep our hands on the body at all times. We can mix-and-match, resting on the body sometimes and hovering over the body at other times during the course of a treatment, and we can do both at the same time: resting one hand on the body while allowing the other hand to hover.

If we are always keeping a hand on the body for fear of losing our 'connection', I wonder what we think that connection is all about.

Distant healing is a standard part of Reiki practice, where you can send the energy to the other side of the planet if we like, just by focusing our attention on the recipient. If we can do that then why would we believe that, at the same time, we can't send Reiki to a person on a treatment couch in front of us – just inches away from us – unless we've made physical contact with them?

It makes no sense at all. 1,000 miles away and sending Reiki's no problem… six inches away and we lose our connection if we're not touching the body. How can that be?

How are we connected?

So what is our Reiki 'connection' to the recipient?

I believe our 'connection' to them is based on our state of mind: by focusing our attention on the recipient we connect to them.

If we think about the Buddhist origins of Reiki and the concept of oneness, there is no 'us' and there is no 'them' anyway: this is illusion! We are already 'connected' to them because in reality we were never separated from them.

We are them.

So, in practice, by being with a client in the same room for the purposes of giving and receiving Reiki, we merge with them, we begin to become one with them. It is our intention that underlies our connection and the energy flows to where our attention is directed, whether our hands are on the body or not.

Over to you

Were you taught that you need to have at least one hand on your client at all times for fear of losing your connection? If so, what has happened in practice? Have you experimented with both-hands-on, one-hand-on and no-hands on?

What feedback have you received from clients where you didn't follow the rules that you were given?

And what do you think about your 'connection' to your client? Do you think it depends on physical contact with them?

Reiki Sensations

In this article I would like to talk about the sort of things that students might feel – or not feel – when receiving attunements or empowerments, when working with energy and when treating or being treated, and the significance of these sensations.

The article is particular addressed to people who have just taken a First Degree course or who are only just starting on their journey with Reiki, though it should be of interest to people at all Reiki levels.

Attunements or empowerments

(Please note that, to avoid unnecessary repetition, I am going to use the word 'empowerment' to refer both to Reiju empowerments and Western-style Reiki attunements.)

When we arrive on a Reiki First Degree course, we probably have very little idea of what we might experience when going through an empowerment. If you read books about Reiki, everyone seems to be going through an exceptional, once-in-a-lifetime experience, but for most people it really isn't like that.

There is no way of predicting what an individual will experience when receiving an empowerment, whether in person or at a distance. You may have an amazing experience, or you may feel very little or nothing. It is not uncommon for people to see some colours or feel some heat or tingling or pulsing or pressure in various areas of their bodies. For some people an empowerment is a unique experience, profound, emotional, an experience that is almost unbelievable. For others very little happens.

Sometimes you might find that there will be four people, say, on a course. Three people are talking about the surprising, or interesting, or special experiences that they just had, and one poor soul is sitting there thinking to themselves "I knew this wouldn't work for me… I know Reiki is supposed to work for everyone, but it hasn't worked for me".

We assume that if we notice a lot happening then the empowerment has 'taken', that it has worked really well, and we assume that if we felt very little – or if we felt nothing – then the connection ritual has not worked, that we haven't been attuned, or we haven't been attuned properly.

But what a student experiences when they receive an empowerment is no guide as to the effectiveness of that empowerment. In fact what a student experiences really is irrelevant, because empowerments always work.

Of course it is nice and reassuring to have the "bells and whistles and fireworks" – it helps you to believe that something definite has happened - but someone who has noticed all these things has not been more effectively empowered when compared with a student who felt very little or nothing.

Experiences are interesting, but not important. They don't mean anything in terms of whether, or how well, an empowerment has worked, because empowerments always work, no matter what the student feels or doesn't feel.

Experiencing energy

People are all different, and people differ in terms of how
sensitive they are to the flow of energy in the early stages of
their work with Reiki. Sometimes people arrive on a Reiki
course massively sensitive to the energy, and perhaps better
able to sense subtle differences than is their teacher, and
that's nice for them, while other people may notice something
very subtle, or perhaps nothing at all. Most people will feel
something.

So when playing with energy, most people will feel something
in between their hands when they try to make an energy ball.
Most people will feel something when they try to feel
someone else's energy field, or if they practise 'scanning'
(assuming that there is something there to detect – there
won't always be). But not everyone will feel these things to
begin with, and the people who do not feel anything should
not be disheartened: because sensitivity to such things can
develop with practice and repetition.

Most people will find that, no matter how sensitive they find
themselves when they first learn Reiki, when they start to
work with the energy regularly – for example by carrying out
Hatsurei ho every day, and by self-treating – their sensitivity
to the energy will increase. But this is a work-in-progress and
we may need to be patient. And we may find that our
sensitivity to the energy never reaches our goal, or is never
as great as other Reiki people that we come across. Maybe
we are setting an unreasonable target for ourselves.

And we should remember that sensitivity to the flow of
energy is not the be-all and end-all of Reiki. We can work on
ourselves and derive the many benefits that come through
Reiki, no matter what we feel or don't feel when we carry out

hatsurei ho or self-treat. We can treat other people effectively no matter what we might feel or not feel in our hands.

I have come across several successful and effective Reiki Master / Teachers who do not feel anything going on in their hands, and never have done. The reason why they continued their Reiki training, rather than giving up in the face of no physical sensations to encourage them, was because they practised on lots of people and they could see, by the positive responses they received from the recipients, that something was definitely going on, that they were doing good things, that Reiki was certainly doing something for the people they treated even though they couldn't feel the energy.

You may ask how you can treat someone when you can't feel anything, or if you can't scan very well at the moment. Well, most people in the world of Reiki are taught a standard set of hand positions to use when they treat, and these standard positions can be followed, giving general coverage over the body; the energy is drawn to areas of need, so that works perfectly well. Not everyone scans.

Not everyone is taught how to scan. It isn't a vital step in a treatment, but it can be a useful one to perform if you can do it.

But if you can work intuitively then of course you can place your hands in the right places for each person you work on, and stay in each position for the most appropriate amount of time, not based on the sensations you are feeling in your hands but based on your intuitive impressions.

Everyone can work intuitively with some practice, and you may well be taught how to carry out "Reiji ho" (a Japanese method for opening to your intuition during a treatment) on a Second Degree course. So an intuitive approach to treatments actually eliminates any advantage in being able to sense strongly in your hands.

Sensations experienced by people you treat

Now, you will not be surprised to know that the experiences of people being treated also varies a great deal. For some people, on some occasions, treatments are very strong. They might feel intense heat from the practitioner's hands, see coloured lights, drift in and out of consciousness. And on other occasions that same person might feel the treatment to be mild and gentle.

The energy is drawn by the recipient in amounts that are appropriate for them on that occasion, so the perceived 'strength' of any treatment is determined by the recipient's need. The practitioner is just a necessary bystander in the treatment process.

While some people seem to quite often notice a lot happening when they are treated, there are also people who feel very little or nothing when they receive a Reiki treatment, no matter who they receive the treatment from.

If you have just started out on your Reiki journey and you just happen to treat one of these people, or a few of these people, as your first 'clients' then you may end up disheartened, thinking that their lack of a strong sensation means that you are ineffective as a practitioner.

We want the recipient to feel a lot because that reassures us that we are doing things 'correctly', that we are effective as a channel for the energy. But things aren't always so simple: while quite often there may be general correlation between what the practitioner feels and what the recipient feels (a very hot area for the practitioner is felt as a very tingly area, say, for the recipient) this correlation will not always be there and, sometimes, you might find a practitioner feeling a raging furnace in their hands, amazed at the strength of what is going on, while the recipient did not notice anything at all, and perhaps didn't notice anything at all during the entire treatment!

Summary

So really this whole article boils down to one simple phrase: "just for today, do not worry". While it is perfectly natural to want to have some physical sensations to help us believe that we are really doing something when we use Reiki on ourselves and on other people, and while most people who learn Reiki will receive sufficient feedback to reassure them, this will not always happen.

With practice and experience we start to let go of the need to be reassured by what we and others feel, and we come to realise that no matter what we feel or don't feel, Reiki is working for us. But it can be difficult to accept this in the early stages, particularly if we are a little sceptical.

If you aren't feeling too much at the moment my advice to you is to follow the instructions you were given: carry out your Hatsurei ho every day, self-treat regularly, and get your hands on as many people as you can.

Do short blasts on someone's knee or shoulder, treat people in a straight-backed chair for 20-30 minutes, do full treatments; go with the time you have you have available.

The important thing is to get the hands-on practice and you will find, if you treat a good cross-section of people, that you will receive from them the positive feedback that you need, and with sufficient practice you may find that you start to notice more with time.

So be patient, don't worry, and have fun with your Reiki.

Treating both sides: is this necessary?

An unnecessary Reiki rule?

In many Reiki lineages, students are taught that they need to treat both sides of a client, asking them to turn over half-way through a treatment so that student can gain access to the client's back. But is this really necessary?

Might the treatment be just as effective if we left them where they were?

I think that most Reiki people would accept that when we treat someone, the energy is drawn according to the recipient's need to the right places for them on that occasion, to do whatever they need to have done on that occasion, so we aren't 'pushing' the energy to where we want it to (or think it ought to) go.

We are a necessary bystander in the process: we need to be there for the healing to happen, but we have metaphorically stepped aside, created a 'healing space' for the client, and they do the healing that they need to do, in the way that they need to do it, experiencing whatever is appropriate for them to experience as this happens.

Could we just hold their hand for 60 minutes?

So, in theory, we could just hold someone's hand for an hour and the energy would be drawn by them to the areas of need, and we'd need to do nothing further than that.

But given that when we work intuitively we can be drawn strongly to areas of need – 'hotspots' – and given that we can experience the flow of energy subsiding in those areas after a time, and given that when we work intuitively we can be guided to hold a series of hand positions, sometimes symmetrical, sometimes not, in a particular sequence, this suggests to me that there is value in allowing the energy to guide you (which is what I believe is happening when you work intuitively), and there is a value in placing your hands in different positions as you treat.

There is something special, I believe, in working in partnership with the energy and allowing it to guide you in terms of where you rest your hands, and for how long you hold each position.

So going through a series of hand positions, whether a set of 'standard' positions or intuitively-guided hand positions, helps to 'fire' the energy from lots of different directions, and it's drawn into the areas that have the greatest need.

We don't just treat the square inches underneath our palms

The energy doesn't just go into a small area of the body underneath our hands when we treat: it moves through the body and you could imagine the energy travelling to chakras, through meridians, into the aura, into all the different aspects of the energy system, physical, mental, emotional, spiritual, whether or not we 'sent' the energy there, because it's being pulled by the recipient's need.

Many of us will have experienced the situation where you're treating one part of the body and the client comments that they can feel the heat, or coldness, or tingling or whatever in a different part of their body.

And because the energy will move from where we 'put it' to where it is needed, this suggests that we do not need to place our hands on every square inch of the body in order for a treatment to be successful, and I do not believe that it is necessary to specifically 'treat' the back in order for the energy to flow to the back of the body from wherever we place our hands.

Turning over routinely is so disruptive

On a practical note, disrupting the flow of a treatment so that the client has to wake up half way through, drag themselves half into the seated position and turn themselves over and get comfortable again, really does break the 'spell' that they are under and, since the relaxation that people experience when receiving Reiki is greatly beneficial, I wouldn't want to wake them up and lessen the depth of their relaxation in this way routinely.

That's not to say that I never treat people's backs, of course.

No rules should be followed slavishly.

But I only do this when someone has a specific back problem and what I do is to start by treating the back for a while, and then turn them over into the 'face-up' treatment position, and carry on with majority of their treatment that way.

In fact, in my First Degree manual I provide a series of hand positions that you can use when treating backs. But I don't recommend that you do that routinely because it's not necessary.

Over to you

If you routinely turn people over half way through a treatment, why not try not doing this and see what happens?

What if I get it wrong?

Getting anxious about our Reiki

When we go on a Reiki course, whether at First Degree, Second Degree or Master Teacher level, we are given instructions telling us how to carry out various tasks, and if we are conscientious then we will try our best to follow those instructions to make sure that we are 'doing it properly'.

So whether we are treating ourselves, giving someone else a Reiki treatment, or performing an attunement on a student, we hope to achieve the desired results by doing it right, by following the instructions to the letter, and if it appears to us that the desired results have not been achieved then we tend to surmise that we have not followed the instructions properly, that we have forgotten something vital and done it wrong, and we may believe that the lack of an expected result is our fault.

If only we could have done things properly then things would have been different.

But there are two problems with this.

Firstly, in reality, not following all the instructions will have very little effect on the efficacy of our treatment or attunement and, secondly, a lack of an expected response or result does not mean that we have done it wrong, or that something has not worked properly.

Treatments that 'go wrong'

Let's think about Reiki treatments for a while.

We have been given a set procedure to follow by our teacher and perhaps we have a certain ritual to carry out before we commence the hands-on treatment. Perhaps we have been given a standard set of hand positions to follow or a set of things that we are 'supposed' to do at the end of a treatment, to bring things to a close.

We carry out the treatment and then the recipient says that they didn't feel very much, or they didn't feel anything at all, or they felt unsettled and not relaxed, and we think back and realise that we missed one of the 'introductory' stages, or we got the words wrong, or we forgot to say something, or we used the 'wrong' sequence of hand positions, or we missed out a hand position or two, or neglected to carry out one of the closing stages of the treatment.

Because the treatment 'didn't work' (apparently) we then assume that this is because we got the treatment wrong, we did the wrong thing, we forgot a vital stage, and it's all our fault.

But we should remind ourselves that not everyone in the world of Reiki is taught to carry out treatments in exactly the same way. Other people may have stages to go through and phrases to say that are very different from how you were taught; they may not have even heard of half the things that you were taught to do, and yet their treatments work perfectly well.

Should we assume that they are not doing things properly because they are not doing it the same way as you?

Or should we assume that your treatment is inadequate because you are missing out vital stages that other people were taught to go through?

Of course not: there are many different ways of approaching giving Reiki treatments, different traditions, different styles, different flavours, some simple, some complex, and they all achieve the desired results.

So we should realise that the 'vital' stages that we were taught to go through are perhaps not quite so vital as we first thought. Reiki accommodates many different ways of working and no phrase or hand movement or ritual is absolutely necessary.

Reiki is above all that fiddly detail

It doesn't matter.

What matters when you treat someone is that you focus your attention on the person you are working on, that you feel yourself merging with the energy and the person in front of you, that you allow yourself to disappear into the energy, neutral, empty, no expectations, and just let it happen.

Anything else beyond that is just frippery, icing on a cake that was fine when it was plain.

We don't need to gild the lily, we don't need to adorn unnecessarily something that was already beautiful, or to make superfluous additions to what is already complete.

So follow the instructions that you were given, by all means, but don't fret if you don't follow the sequence exactly, and please allow yourself the freedom to tailor your routine according to what feels right for you; find your own style and comfortable way of working rather than slavishly following a set of instructions passed on to you by another person.

Go with what feels right for you on that occasion; be guided by intuition.

And why should we assume that the treatment did not work, that the session did not give the recipient what they needed, just because they felt very little, or felt nothing happening, or felt unrelaxed during the treatment? While many people have a wonderful time while being treated, seeing coloured lights, feeling tingling sensations or intense heat from the practitioner's hands, experiencing deep relaxation and peace, melting into the treatment table, not everyone experiences that.

Not everyone is the same.

Not all recipients have a great time when they receive Reiki. Some people feel nothing, some feel very little, and some are quite unsettled by the whole experience. But no matter what they noticed happening, they received what they needed, and they experienced whatever sensations they needed to experience.

It's nice to have positive feedback at the end of a treatment session, and people saying how relaxed they were and how hot our hands were etc. helps to boost our confidence, but such things are not compulsory and not everyone will say these things. We didn't mess up their treatment because it would be very difficult to mess up a Reiki treatment: Reiki is foolproof!

Attunements that 'go wrong'

The same comments apply to the carrying out of attunements.

There are very many different attunement styles being used in the world, some quite simple, some quite complicated, and there will be stages and ritual movements or phrases/affirmations being used by some teachers that are not being used all by other teachers.

One teacher may be going through – to them – a vital stage that others do not replicate, while others will be doing 'necessary' practices that we do not follow. And yet all these attunement styles work.

So while we should always try and do our best, and follow the attunement instructions that we were given, we should not worry terribly if we realise that we have missed out a particular stage or forgot to say a particular phrase, or failed to draw a symbol perfectly.

What is important when attuning someone is your underlying intent; the details of the ritual are there to create a ritual 'space' in which the attunement can occur, but there are no really vital stages that have to be carried out no matter what, so we should not worry.

And we should remember that the reaction of a student to an attunement will vary greatly.

If a student feels very little or nothing we should not assume that the attunement has not 'taken'; this would not be possible. Equally, we should not assume that a student who experienced 'bells and whistles' has been far more effectively attuned. Such sensations and experiences are nice for the recipient but do not really indicate anything significant.

Attunements work, even with some mistakes, and sometimes the recipient has an amazing experience; sometimes not.

It doesn't matter what they feel or don't feel.

Chill out, Dude!

So we should feel confident that Reiki is giving the recipient what they need, whether they are receiving a treatment or an attunement, we should try our best and be conscientious but we should not worry too much if we don't follow all the instructions.

We should allow ourselves to find our own style, own comfortable way of working, which may be a little different from other people's but which is just as valid, and we should not assume that a lack of 'bells and whistles' on the part of the recipient means that something hasn't happened.

There is no one 'correct' way to do things, there is no correct response to treatments or attunements, and Reiki accommodates many different styles and approaches.

So we can relax!

Declutter your treatment rituals

Time for a Reiki spring clean?

Reiki treatments are carried out in a lot of different ways and many rituals have been developed and passed on in different lineages.

Reiki has also been affected by the belief systems of people who are involved in other energy practices and it's natural for Reiki teachings to become 'coloured' by a teacher's personal quirks and idiosyncrasies too.

Trouble is, these practices end up turning into "this is the way that you have to do it" as they are passed on from teacher to student, teacher to new teacher, and that's unfortunate since some people end up lumbered with quite complex rituals that they feel they have to carry out for a treatment to be done 'properly'.

Reiki is greater than that.

Reiki works simply and intuitively and doesn't need to be accompanied by a lot of dogma. There will be Reiki practitioners out there who treat their clients using a lot of rituals that other effective Reiki practitioners do not use, and there will be people out there using Reiki effectively while not carrying out stages and rituals that other practitioners regard as essential.

Let's look at a few examples of ideas and practices that I regard as unnecessary.

If you were taught to do these things, why not experiment and find your own approach.

Keep at least one hand on the body at all times for fear of losing your connection

I have written about this one before, and if we can send Reiki from one side of the planet to the other just by thinking of someone, there will be no problem in 'losing' your connection to a client on a treatment table in front of you should your hands stray a few inches from their body.

'Connection' is a state of mind and comes through focusing your attention on the recipient. If you're doing a Reiki treatment on someone then you are connected to them!

Treat from head to toe and then you must go back up the body from feet to head

Seems a bit clumsy to me, and is sometimes combined with the previous paragraph, so you end up with "always keep at least one hand on the body at all times and work from head to foot, and then back to the head again".

The general approach within Reiki seems to be to work from head to feet, though working the other way might be the right thing to do sometimes.

My approach is to work intuitively so I don't follow a set of rules that have to be applied to every client in the same way. Why should every client receive the same format of treatment? They have different problems, different energy needs.

'One size fits all' doesn't fit very well with me.

Always throw out 'negative' energy at the end of treatment

If you believe that there is negative energy and if you believe that it will stay with the client (and presumably cause them problems) if you don't throw it away, then I suppose you'd better throw it away.

And if you've got it on you before you throw it away then presumably you don't want that stuff hanging around on you either, so you really need to throw it away.

But not everyone is taught that and not everyone does that, and some people believe that Reiki is a pure healing energy that is drawn by the recipient's need, and gives the recipient what they need on that occasion, balancing and transforming in a way that is right for them.

And in that case, we wouldn't need to think in terms of accumulating stuff that Reiki couldn't get rid of, and dealing with it ourselves.

Always 'ground' the energy at the end of a treatment by putting your hands on the floor

Some people do seem to have quite a bee in their bonnet on the issue of grounding.

They put almost every malady down to not being grounded, and have their students frantically grounding themselves.

On a personal level, grounding is easy: go for a walk, do the washing up, breathe in some fresh air and you're grounded. Hatsurei ho – daily energy exercises – grounds you.

I believe that giving a Reiki treatment is a grounding exercise.

So what is this ungrounded energy that you have to deal with when you put your hands on the floor – is it your energy, is it the client's "ungrounded" energy, and what would happen if you didn't crouch down and touch the floorboards?

Isn't Reiki a bit more effective than that?

Does it really need us to come along and sort out stuff that it hasn't dealt with properly?

Recite a set of words at the start of a treatment that 'have' to be said

Many people have a set form of words that they say to themselves to get them in the right frame of mind for carrying out a Reiki treatment, and I have no problem with that.

This can be useful and helpful.

But some people are taught that "these words are THE words" that you have to say at the start of the treatment, with the corollary that if you haven't said them, or if you mess up the words, then the treatment's not going to go properly.

If you've said a set of words time and again before starting a treatment, don't you think your subconscious mind knows what it's all about, and that you have that intention 'programmed' into you already?

Intention is a very important thing with Reiki and I don't think you need to keep on reminding and re-reminding yourself about what you want to happen.

Over to you

I hope the above comments have provided some food for thought and if you are currently using the practices described above, why not try a different approach, see what happens, and come to your own conclusions about what's the best way for you to approach treating others.

Have you altered your own approach compared to what you were originally taught, and have you found that leaving behind some of those rules and restrictions has been fine?

Reiki treatments and winning the lottery

Let's talk about cause and effect

Sometimes I am asked by my students about things that happen to a client after they have had a Reiki treatment. The questions are usually framed in terms of:

"After the treatment, this happened... is that the Reiki?"

"I gave someone a treatment and the next week *x* happened... was that the Reiki?"

Sometimes my response is [shrugs shoulders]... maybe, or "who knows"... sometimes I will say "probably" or "could be".

And that's about as far as I can go because (1) I don't have a crystal ball and (2) not everything that happens to a person after they have had a Reiki treatment, or been on a Reiki course, is a result of the Reiki that they received or were initiated into.

Reiki and the lottery

So someone goes on a Reiki course and the next week they win the lottery. Is Reiki responsible for this? Has the universe conspired in such a way as to bring that person their winning numbers because they decided to learn Reiki?

Someone has a Reiki treatment and the next week they get run over by a 'bus. Is the Reiki responsible for this event?

The answer is no: not everything that happens to a person after Reiki is because of the Reiki.

Because things occur randomly: unusual things happen to people sometimes, things appear out of the blue.

And because we seek to fnd an explanation for the things that happen to us in our lives, we try and attach that happening to something, something different or new that we have done or experienced.

How do we know whether something was because of the Reiki?

You don't.

Not in an individual case.

You can only look at a group of people and see what sort of things they tend to experience after receiving or learning Reiki, and you can find themes emerging, experiences or happenings that seem to turn up again and again and again.

And then when that happens to another student, you can say, "yes, that probably was the Reiki", but you'll never know absolutely definitely because the thing they are reporting may have just happened anyway.

So what does Reiki do for people then?

Whether you receive a course of treatments or if you are learning Reiki for yourself, you should find that Reiki helps you to feel more 'laid back' – calm, content and serene – and you should find that you feel better able to deal with stressful situations or stressful people, and that you feel more positive and better able to cope.

If energy levels are low then they can be boosted; if spirits are low then they can be lifted.

This 'Reiki effect' seems to be noticed in most people who learn Reiki and work on themselves regularly, or in people who receive a course of Reiki treatments.

The decluttering effect

One of the things that I have noticed, based on my experiences when teaching students through my Reiki Home Study courses, is the "decluttering" effect that Reiki can have on many people.

Reiki seems to cause people to want, or to find, a simpler way through their life, and that can involve ditching things: ditching household clutter, ditching unwanted commitments and habits, clearing out cupboards and spare rooms, simplifying your life on lots of levels.

Over to you

So, what things have you experienced as a result of receiving Reiki treatments that you are fairly certain are because of the Reiki?

What changes occurred in your life after you learned Reiki that you're fairly sure are because of the system that you learned?

How has Reiki changed things for the better for you?

Reiki is not all fluffy bunnies!

When Reiki shifts up a gear

We know what Reiki tends to do for people, don't we? People end up chilled, calm, serene, content, better able to cope, more positive.

Reiki brings balance, perspective, and if you add in a regular focus on the Reiki precepts, and the practise of mindfulness, then you have a really powerful system for positive change.

But it's not all happy bunnies and smiles: Reiki can produce powerful effects and elicit powerful shifts in a person.

When someone comes for a Reiki treatment, they will usually have a wonderful experience. They will feel more relaxed than they have for a very long time, they will drift, or float, or sink, they will bliss out on those boiling hot hands, they might have rainbow light shows, or tingles, a lovely experience.

But it's not like that for everyone.

Sometimes a person can just feel generally 'unsettled' during a treatment. They don't relax, they don't necessarily experience anything powerful, but they're not calm and relaxed and peaceful, as most people are. So what is going on here?

Well, they are having a definite experience, the energy is doing something for them, and what it is doing is coming through as that sense of being unsettled.

The energy will provide the recipient with a variety of sensations or feelings, and they are just what that person needs to experience to best shift what they need to shift to move on, a side-effect, in a way, of the energetic work that is going on within them.

Often it's a lovely experience, but not always.

Emotional shifts

Sometimes Reiki can produce powerful emotional effects in a short space of time, as people release what they need to release to move on with their lives.

It's as if all this deeply-embedded stuff is bubbling to the surface to be released.

So I have had people literally wailing on the treatment table, and it's not uncommon to see a silent tear or two pass from someone's eye as they're treated.

And although it's not nice to see someone in distress, it seems that these emotions, although powerful at times, are experienced in a positive way by the client, where there is a sense of relief that they are just letting go, moving on from what they are experiencing on the treatment table.

So don't worry if someone becomes emotional when you treat them. This is common. It shows that things are moving, shifting, and that's what you and your client want.

By the end of the session, everything will have calmed down and your client will feel much better. The treatment will have come like a breath fo fresh air, like a cleansing breath that has flushed out accumulated gunk.

And while your client may sometimes feel a bit shell-shocked by what they experienced, they will have left stuff behind and moved on in some positive fashion.

Physical shifts

While the 'emotional release' is probably more common than its physical counterpart, sometimes a client will experience more physical sensations, for example pain. It's not uncommon for someone with arthritis, for example, to experience a short-term intensification of those joint pains, while they are receiving their treatment, though the pains then subside and often improve subsequently.

I have treated people with metal plates inserted into their bones, where the area has ached during a treatment, for example.

Aftershocks

A Reiki treatment is rather like dropping a pebble into a pond: while there is the initial splash, during the treatment – an intensification of things – the energy will also produce ripples that carry on, with peaks and troughs.

So it's not uncommon for a client to experience some emotional ups and downs in the days after a treatment, with physical effects like better sleep, or disturbed sleep, aches and pains, feeling full of energy, or feeling tired and wanting to change gear and slow down for a while.

These things are all side-effects of the energy working to bring things into balance for that person, giving them the opportunity to re-balance, to reinterpret, to reconsider, to achieve a new state of wellness.

Over to you

What powerful effects have you or witnessed when giving a Reiki treatment? What did your client experience and how did that help them to improve things subsequently?

What have you experienced for yourself when receiving a Reiki treatment that would consider to be a powerful experience, and how has that helped you?

The Kaizen of Reiki

If you have come across the word 'kaizen' before it will probably have been in the context of industrial quality control or personal development.

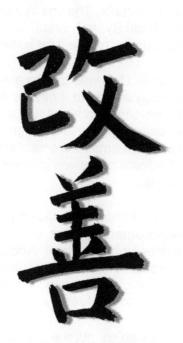

"Kaizen" is a Japanese word that is usually translated as 'improvement', but it means more than that. The word has connotations of continuous, gradual, orderly and never-ending improvement, the willingness to constantly, relentlessly pursue improvement a small step at a time.

The application of the kaizen principle is the reason why Japan's economy was transformed after the Second World War. All workers were encouraged to make suggestions as to how quality and production could be improved, even by tiny, tiny percentages, but over time the effect of these tiny percentage improvements, applied consistently and built upon, transformed Japanese industry.

So what has this to do with Reiki?

"Kaizen" is in the Reiki precepts

Well the word kaizen actually appears towards the end of the
Reiki precepts. The line in Japanese is "Shin shin kaizen,
Usui Reiki Ryoho", which could be loosely translated as
"Mind body change it for better Usui Reiki method".

So when Usui was talking about using his system to improve
the body and mind, I get the impression that we are looking
at a lifelong commitment to work with the system, to focus
the energy on ourselves again and again, long-term, in order
to produce small incremental improvements within ourselves,
to dedicate ourselves to developing our effectiveness as a
channel.

But small changes build on previous small changes, an
enhancement upon an enhancement leads to amazing
development over time. And Usui's original system gives us
the solid, concrete techniques that we can use to develop
ourselves: as channels, in terms of spirituality and in terms of
intuition, to produce our own individual Reiki Evolution!

So how do we pursue our own kaizen of Reiki? How do we
apply the concept of continuous and never-ending
improvement to our practice of Reiki? Here are a few
suggestions…

Root your practice of Reiki in daily energy work.

If you are serious about wanting to obtain the many benefits
that are available to you through the Reiki system then you
are going to have to work on yourself most days, ideally
every day, and by doing so you will build up the beneficial
effects of Reiki within you.

It is not sufficient to use Reiki on yourself once a week, or to assume that if you treat other people occasionally then this is enough to give you the Reiki you need.

Your first priority should be yourself, and this means daily energy work.

This does not need to be an onerous task, nor does it need to take a long time to carry out. Sometimes we decline to use Reiki on ourselves because we do not have the perfect opportunity, perhaps because we do not have, say, 30 minutes to work on ourselves.

Yet even 10 minutes of energy work, when carried out consistently each day, would be far better and produce much better results than doing nothing for days, and then a great big blitz for a big chunk of time on a weekend to try and 'catch up'.

Spending even a small chunk of time working on ourselves each day builds up a momentum and stirs changes which build and build.

Sporadic practice leads to some beneficial changes, but you are not maximising your Reiki potential.

So, how can we work on ourselves?

Well, a good place to start would be to practise Hatsurei ho, a series of energy exercises taught in the Usui Reiki Ryoho Gakkai (the 'Gakkai), an association set up after Usui's death by the Imperial Officers who had trained with him for a while.

'Hatsurei ho' means something like 'start up Reiki technique' and consists of a series of energy meditations/ visualisations that focus on your Tanden (Dantien in Chinese) and which are designed to be carried out every day.

The effects of Hatsurei ho are to:

1. Clear and cleanse your energy system
2. Help to move your energy system more into a state of balance
3. Help to ground you
4. Help to build up your personal energy reserves
5. Allows you to grow spiritually
6. Develop your ability as a channel for Reiki
7. Help to develop your sensitivity to the flow of energy
8. Help to develop your intuitive side

The exercises take perhaps 12-15 minutes to carry out each day, and can be fitted into the busiest of schedules if the will is there. We can all make this time for our Reiki practice.

But we should also focus the energy more specifically on ourselves, on our own self-healing, by carrying out a self-treatment each day.

Whether you carry out the Western 'hands-on' method of treating yourself, or use the self-treatment meditation that Usui Sensei taught, you should focus the energy on yourself on a regular basis to help bring things into balance for you on all levels, and to help you to release things that no longer serve you: mental states, emotions, physical things.

The energy will deal with many aspects of your body/mind, many deeply-embedded imbalances, if we give the energy the opportunity to do its work on us, digging deep and chipping away at the 'baggage' that we carry, over time.

We prefer to use Usui Sensei's self-treatment meditation because it seems more intense and versatile, but all self-treatment approaches are valid. Usui's Sensei's system was all about spiritual development and self-healing, so Hatsurei Ho and self-treatment can lie at the very heart of your Reiki practice.

You need to put yourself first, and the principle of kaizen means that by working on yourself consistently, great transformations are possible. You owe it to yourself to allow yourself to obtain the benefits that are available to you through Reiki.

Receive spiritual empowerments throughout your training and beyond.

Training with Usui was rather like martial arts training, where you were in ongoing contact with your teacher over an extended period of time. Part of your training involved receiving simple spiritual empowerments from Usui Sensei, repeatedly, at all levels.

Each empowerment reinforced your connection to the source, cleared your channel for the energy, allowed you to develop spiritually and enhanced your intuitive potential.

To echo this practice, Taggart sends out a distant Reiju empowerment every week, on a Monday, which can be 'tuned in to' by any Reiki person.

You can find out about this, and what to do, by visiting the Reiki Evolution web site.

On each occasion that you receive Reiju you are given what you need, and as your needs change from one occasion to another, this simple spiritual 'blessing' helps you to develop. A one-off attunement or empowerment does of course give you something permanent, and when you learn Reiki for the first time the attunements or empowerments that you receive provide you with the ability to use Reiki permanently, but it does not stop there: by receiving empowerments on a regular basis you are building momentum and allowing the energy to penetrate more deeply within you.

If we are committed to ongoing improvements within ourselves then we should make the time to receive an empowerment weekly. And again it is the regular commitment which is the key, the key to deepening your experience of the energy and its beneficial effects on you.

Work on developing your intuitive potential.

Mikao Usui's original system did not focus very much on the treatment of others, and any instruction on treatments would not have involved slavishly following a set of 'standard' hand positions that you had to apply to everyone you treated. Usui's method was simpler and more elegant. You allowed the energy to guide your hands to the right place to treat, different from one person to another, and different within the same person from one treatment to another.

The way we have been taught to do this is through a 'technique' called 'Reiji Ho' (indication of the spirit technique'), a way of emptying your mind and merging with the energy, getting your head out of the way to allow intuition to bubble to the surface.

The exciting thing about Reiji Ho is that it works for everyone, and with time - we come back to kaizen's small incremental improvements - your hands will move more quickly, more consistently, more effortlessly, and you will start to attract more intuitive information. So every time we treat someone we should spend time cultivating our 'Reiji' state of mind, and gradually, gradually, we develop.

Learn to become the energies.

…that you are introduced to at Second Degree and Master levels. Usui's system didn't involve symbols as far as most of his students were concerned. Students were expected to carry out meditations over an extended period of time in order to learn to experience different energies and, at Second Degree, students were introduced to the energies of "earth ki" and "heavenly ki", which represent two fundamental aspects of our being.

By practising 'becoming' earth ki and heavenly ki again and again – a powerful self-healing practice - these energies became so familiar to the students that they could 'connect' to the energy direct without having to use a prop like a symbol.

Usui provided some Shinto mantras for some of his students to use to invoke the energies, but it was possible to move beyond these mantras with time, too. In my article 'A Simple Way with Symbols' I describe a meditation that you can use to 'become' these energies.

But again we see that to obtain the greatest benefit, to enhance self-healing, to free up our practice and move beyond symbols, takes time and commitment. A quick meditation carried out a few times is not enough: Usui Sensei's students spent 6-9 months meditating on just one energy, and this was done because the principle of kaizen – plugging away and developing by small amounts again and again – led to deep changes over time.

Live your life according to Usui's guiding principles.

Usui's simple principles to live by offer perhaps the best example of the principle of kaizen in our Reiki practice: Usui Sensei's precepts are a work in progress. They are not something that you read through and think "OK, got that": the precepts are simple to read and understand but they are something that you drip-feed into your daily life over time, more and more over time.

We may begin by thinking about the precepts when we first come across them on a First Degree course: we reflect on how they might impinge on our lives, our thoughts and emotions, our behaviour; we might imagine situations from that past that might have proceeded better had we exemplified the precepts, and we might imagine situations in the future and see ourselves behaving in a way that demonstrates that we are living the precepts.

But this initial surge of interest in the precepts is not sufficient to produce the beneficial changes that the precepts can produce in our lives.

To fully embrace Usui Sensei's spiritual principles takes regular reflection and ongoing thought. On an ongoing basis we consider our thoughts and our behaviour, we reflect on the principles and what they mean to us.

If we do this then over time we will find that living the precepts becomes easier, that our behaviour is modifying itself, that there are more permanent changes in the way that we react and behave and relate to other people. But this will only happen if we 'chip away' at our current behaviour patterns, using the precepts as our guiding light. There are no quick fixes: the precepts are not just for First Degree. The precepts are the essence of our Reiki practice.

Now, we do not need to be perfect, we do not need to beat ourselves up for not applying each and every principle on all occasions, but by dedicating ourselves, and by forgiving ourselves, and by trying to do a little better each day than we did the day before, we transform ourselves.

That is the key to our kaizen of Reiki: dedication and commitment, patience and forgiveness, and openness to the source.

Long term.

Get out of the way!

In this short article I want to talk about the best way to approach working on other people, whether giving treatments or carrying out distant healing. I want to talk about our state of mind and our intent when channelling the energy.

The first thing I want to say is that we are just a channel for the energy, not the source of the energy. This seems an obvious thing to say, but we need to remember that we are not healers. We do not heal. We do not have that power.

What we do when we treat someone is simply to create a 'healing space' that the recipient can use to move more into a state of balance. The recipient is responsible for their own healing, for what they experience or don't experience; they are responsible for how they react to the treatment. They are healing themselves.

"Necessary bystanders"

We are just necessary bystanders in the process: we do not direct the energy and we do not determine the outcome.

So I am not so happy with the title "Reiki Healer" because it suggests that the Reiki practitioner has the power to heal; they do not. I don't think that the title "Reiki Necessary Bystander" is going to catch on, so I prefer to use the title "Reiki Practitioner". It describes what we do: we practise Reiki and it does not imply that we have the power to heal others.

This article is called "Get out of the way" because I believe that this is the best thing we can do when treating someone or when sending distant healing. We are not the source of the healing; we are not the source of the energy, so we do not need to be there, directing and controlling. We can stand aside and if we do so then the energy can flow strongly and clearly, without interference from us.

When we treat someone we are not 'cheerleading' for a particular end result: we do not give Reiki to get rid of someone's head ache, or back ache, or to resolve their Gall Bladder problem, though of course these things may result from channelling Reiki.

End results are out of our hands and to focus strongly on a particular purpose for the treatment is not helpful. Reiki will not be controlled by us in terms of end results and attempts to control the energy in this way just puts up barriers that prevent the energy from doing what it needs to do.

Rather like the well-meaning amateur who gets in the way and prevents the professional from doing their job properly, our attempts to focus the energy to produce a particular end result will hinder the process for the recipient.

Having a neutral intent

So our intent when treating someone or sending distant healing is that the energy should do whatever is appropriate for the recipient. We are neutral, we are detached, and we do not focus on outcomes. Ideally we should drift into a gentle meditative state when treating or sending distant healing, and this can be best achieved by our 'disappearing' into the energy, feeling ourselves merging with or becoming one with the energy.

We merge with the energy and we merge with the recipient; we are empty. We do by not doing.

Giving treatments while distracted

Though some people are taught that it is ok to talk and chat to people, or bystanders, when giving a Reiki treatment, to do such a thing is neither professional nor does it lead to effective treatments.

If we are distracted then the energy flows less strongly, so if we want to do the best for our clients then we need to keep quiet, and encourage the client to keep quiet too. You can try an experiment for yourself if you like, to prove to yourself that distraction lessens the strength of your Reiki.

You could try this at a Reiki share, for example. Start by resting your hands on someone's shoulders and allow the energy to flow for a while. Then deliberately start up a conversation with someone sitting near you: take your attention away from the recipient and fully engage in the conversation. Do this for a few minutes. Then bring your attention back to the recipient, be still and quiet, and allow the energy to flow. How has the recipient's experience of the energy varied?

Now, we do not need to be in a perfect meditative state in order to be an effective channel for Reiki, but it certainly helps to cultivate a still and empty mind. We are all human and it is perfectly normal for unwanted thoughts to appear in our head. But we should pay them no attention.

If we pay the unwanted thoughts attention and try to get rid of them we then have two lots of thoughts: the thoughts we did not want and all the new thoughts about the need to get rid of the first lot of thoughts. We have made things worse!

The best approach to unwanted thoughts, then, is to allow them to drift by like clouds: pay them no attention, do not engage with them. They will leave.

Some more may come, but pay them no attention either. In time you should find that your busy mind starts to quieten and some of your treatments will become beautiful meditations, with your mind emptying with the energy, and staying empty.

Some treatments will not be like this, of course, but we do not need to be perfect. We can cultivate a more meditative state over time, moving in the right direction, and without worrying too much about individual occasions when our untamed brain kept on talking to us. This is a work-in-progress!

So Reiki is simple: you empty your head, you merge with the energy, do you not direct, you do not control, you do not try; you empty yourself and merge with the recipient, standing aside to allow the energy do what it needs to do, without interference from us.

Reiki advice from Bruce Lee: Be like water

Excellent advice

"Be formless, shapeless... like water"

"True refinement seeks simplicity"

You might be surprised to hear that these words were spoken by Bruce Lee, film star and famous martial artist who developed Jeet Kune Do, a hybrid martial arts method that took the best approaches from different fighting systems and synthesised them into a flexible and effective fighting art.

Jeet Kune Do is referred to as a "style without style" where, unlike more traditional martial arts which Lee saw as rigid and formalistic, JKD is not fixed or patterned: it is more of a philosophy with guiding thoughts, a "style of no style". Bruce Lee often referred to JKD as "The art of expressing the human body" in his writings and in interviews.

And those comments got me wondering about Reiki, especially when Lee identified three different stages that someone's practice could go through.

He said that before training, people had a natural ability, something that was unformed and unfocused; training begins and the student learns how to follow the instruction, they are restricted to the framework that they are taught and many practitioners might not move beyond that stage, following the system almost by rote.

The third stage is where the practitioner moves beyond the rote learning to embrace simplicity and flexibility.

So how does that echo one's development with Reiki?

Well, before some people learn Reiki, they already have a healing ability, maybe unstructured or unconscious, unfocused, but a natural healing ability nevertheless. We have taught many such people, who have found that Reiki gives them a framework or a structure to work through, focusing and channelling and enhancing what they already had.

The student learns a particular approach, with some rules and standard hand positions and in some lineages quite a long list of things you can and can't, should and shouldn't, do with Reiki. Some practitioners remain at this stage, following the instructions they were given and remaining content with that way of working.

But you can move beyond that framework, simplifying your practice, altering what you do to the needs of the recipient.

You can embrace intuitive working, where you leave behind those basic rules to go 'freestyle' and, where Lee describes his system as "The art of expressing the human body", we could see intuitive working as "The art of expressing the energy".

Here we are empty and formless, flowing like water to where the water wants to go, joining with the energy and following it, directing the energy to where it wants to be directed, emphasising aspects of the energy that need to be emphasised.

We stand as a flexible conduit between the source and the recipient, empty, formless, fluid.

I believe that clutter-free Reiki is the best Reiki, and that by cutting away the rules and the dogma we can 'refine' (to use Lee's word) our Reiki practice.

Emptiness is the goal

Emptiness is the goal here: no planning, no thought about what you might do, just being there with the energy and the recipient; your treatment has no form, no structure and you simply follow the flow of energy, becoming the energy, merging with the recipient, with no expectations other than to just 'be'.

Over to you

Can you see Bruce Lee's description of advancement within martial arts in your own practice of Reiki?

Have you moved on from the basic procedures that you were taught, to find your own comfortable way with the energy?

Has Bruce Lee's advice that you should be "Be formless, shapeless... like water" and that "True refinement seeks simplicity" insinuated itself into the way that you practise Reiki now?

Simple energy exercises to get the energy flowing

In this post I'd like to share a couple of simple Reiki energy exercises that you can use to clear and cleanse, and balance your energy system. These exercises come from Original Japanese Reiki, were taught by Mikao Usui, and can be used every day.

They would be a lovely way to start your day, in fact.

The exercises are referred to as **kenyoku**, which means "dry bathing" and **joshin kokkyu ho**, which means something like "soul cleansing breathing method". You carry out the exercises in order, starting with a quick kenyoku and then moving on to a blissful experience when carrying out joshin kokkyu ho for several minutes.

Here's what to do:

Relax

Sit in a comfortable chair. Relax and close your eyes, and place your hands palms down on your lap.

Focus your attention on your Dantien point: an energy centre two fingerbreadths (3-5 cm) below your tummy button and 1/3 of the way into your body.

Say to yourself "I'm starting my energy exercises now".

Kenyoku

Kenyoku can be seen as a way of getting rid of negative energy.

Brush across your torso

Place the fingertips of your right hand near the top of the left shoulder, where the collarbone meets the bulge of the shoulder. The hand is lying flat on your chest. Draw your flat hand down and across the chest in a straight line, over the base of the sternum (where your breastbone stops and your abdomen starts, in the midline) and down to the right hip.

Exhale as you do this.

Do the same on the right side, using your left hand. Draw your left hand from the right shoulder, in a straight line across the sternum, to the left hip, and again exhale as you make the downward movement.

Do the same on the left side again (like you did at the start), so you will have carried out movements with your right hand, left hand, and right hand again.

Brush down your arms

Now put your right fingertips on the outer edge of the left shoulder, at the top of your slightly outstretched left arm, with your fingertips pointing sideways away from your body.

Move your right hand, flattened, along the outside of your arm, all the way to the fingertips and beyond, all the while keeping the left arm straight. Exhale as you do this.

130

Repeat this process on the right side, with the left hand placed on the right shoulder, and move it down the right arm to the fingertips and beyond. Exhale as you do this.

Repeat the process on the left side again, so you will have carried out movements with your right hand, left hand, and right hand again, like before.

Once you have carried out kenyoku, move straight on to joshin kokkyu ho.

Joshin kokkyu ho

Joshin kokkyu ho means 'Technique for Purification of the Spirit' or 'Soul Cleansing Breathing Method'. It is a meditation that focuses on the Dantien point.

Put your hands on your lap with your palms facing upwards and breathe naturally through your nose. Do not overbreathe: breathe naturally and gently.

Focus on your Dantien point and relax.

When you breathe in, visualise energy or light flooding into your crown chakra and passing into your Dantien and, as you pause before exhaling, feel that energy expand throughout your body, melting all your tensions.

When you breathe out, imagine that the energy floods out of your body in all directions as far as infinity.

Get into a nice gentle even rhythm of drawing the energy down, spreading it through your body, and flooding it out to the universe.

Do this for 10-15 minutes. You may feel energy/tingling in your hands and even in your feet, as the meditation progresses, but don't worry if you don't, because everyone is different.

Over to you

Carry out this sequence every day for a couple of weeks and notice what difference it makes to you in terms of:

- The strength of the energy
- Your sensitivity to the energy
- Your general contentment or demeanour

Have fun!

The simplest self-treatment meditation ever!

How were you taught to Self-Treat?

Most people who are taught Reiki will have been taught some form of self-treatment, a way of focusing the energy on yourself, for your own benefit, and the most common form of self-treatment is what I would refer to as a "Standard Western hands-on" self-treatment method.

This is where you rest your hands in a series of positions covering the head and torso and maybe beyond, and let the energy flow out of your hands into your body.

It works well, though some of the positions can often be uncomfortable to get to, or hold for any amount of time, and that can often detract from the blissfulness of the experience.

So what I'm going to talk about in a series of articles are "how to do Reiki on yourself" in a number of different ways, ways to Reiki self-treat that are perhaps different from what you have been taught.

And I'd like to start with what you might call "The simplest self-treatment method ever"!

Taggart's "Meditation with the intention to heal"

It is possible to self-treat without resting your hands on your body at all, using your intention or visualisation or pure intent. In this example, what you are doing is, basically, setting a definite intent and letting the energy do what it wants to do.

Here are some instructions:

- Make yourself comfortable in a seated position, maybe with your hands resting in your lap
- Close your eyes
- Start to become aware of your connection to the energy, your connection to Reiki
- Notice how that connection feels, with the energy engulfing you and building within you in just the right way for you in this moment
- As the energy flows, just remind yourself that your intention now is to heal, to heal on all levels, to rejuvenate, to rebalance
- Just say to yourself, "this is my time to heal now"
- And allow the energy to flow, to flow to wherever it needs to go to give you just what you need in this moment
- Stay in this safe space, allowing the energy to provide balance, and healing
- And finally bring yourself back when you feel ready, and open your eyes

So this method doesn't involve hand positions, or symbols, it doesn't require visualisation, it doesn't direct the energy in any way. You sit, you merge with the energy and you allow it to flow, to do what it needs to do.

And you can just be there as a bystander in the process, observing, experiencing, in a neutral way: merged with the energy.

Over to you

If this self-treatment method is new to you, why not give it a try?

Intuitive self-healing meditation

Taggart's "Intuitive self-healing meditation"

This is still a very simple self-treatment method, where you're not resting your hands on yourself, but allowing the self-healing to occur through meditating.

What is new in this meditation is that we are going is to notice where the energy is flowing, and we are going to focus our attention on those areas.

Here's what to do.

- Make yourself comfortable in a seated position, maybe with your hands resting in your lap, and close your eyes
- Start to become aware of your connection to the energy, your connection to Reiki
- Notice how that connection feels, with the energy engulfing you and building within you in just the right way for you in this moment
- As the energy flows, just remind yourself that your intention now is to heal, to heal on all levels, to rejuvenate, to rebalance
- Just say to yourself, "this is my time to heal now"
- And allow the energy to flow, to flow to wherever it needs to go to give you just what you need in this moment
- ***And start to become aware of the energy and where it's flowing***

- *Where is the Reiki focusing itself, where is it dwelling?*
- *Allow your attention to rest on that area; bring your awareness there*
- *If the energy moves on to another area, bring your attention to that new area, and notice the energy there*
- Stay in this safe space, allowing the energy to provide balance, and healing
- And finally bring yourself back when you feel ready, and open your eyes

So this method doesn't involve hand positions, or symbols, it doesn't require visualisation, it doesn't direct the energy in any way. You sit, you merge with the energy and you allow it to flow, to do what it needs to do.

What is different, though, is your attention: you follow the flow of energy and wherever the energy is directing itself, you focus your attention there too.

This is a powerful thing to do because where you focus your attention is where the energy focuses itself.

By allowing your attention to rest on the areas of need, you intensify and boost the flow of energy because "where thought goes, energy flows".

And you can just be there as a bystander in the process, observing, experiencing, in a neutral way: merged with the energy and following the flow of energy.

Over to you

If this self-treatment method is new to you, why not give it a try?

Mikao Usui's original self-treatment meditation

In my last article I described my "intuitive Reiki self-healing meditation" where you followed the flow of energy and focused your attention on the areas where the energy wanted to go.

This was a beneficial practice because resting your attention somewhere helps to boost the flow of Reiki, making the treatment more intense and focused in the areas that your attention is dwelling on.

So now we can build on the idea of the energy focusing itself where your attention is dwelling, by carrying out a meditation where you allow your attention to rest on five different areas of the head, spending a few minutes focusing on each position. This is a self-treatment method taught by Reiki's founder, Mikao Usui.

The Usui self-treatment meditation

Here's what to do.

- Make yourself comfortable in a seated position, maybe with your hands resting in your lap, and close your eyes
- Start to become aware of your connection to the energy, your connection to Reiki
- Notice how that connection feels, with the energy engulfing you and building within you in just the right way for you in this moment

- As the energy flows, just remind yourself that your intention now is to heal, to heal on all levels, to rejuvenate, to rebalance
- Just say to yourself, "this is my time to heal now"
- *Allow your attention to focus on your forehead, by the hairline, and allow the energy to dwell there, building, intensifying*
- *Move your attention so you focus on your temples, on both sides of your head at the same time*
- *Move your attention so that you focus on the back of the head, and on the forehead, those two areas at the same time*
- *Move your focus so your attention comes to rest on the back of your neck, the base of your skull*
- *Move your attention to the crown, the crown of your head, focus your attention there*
- And finally bring yourself back when you feel ready, and open your eyes

So this method doesn't involve physical hand positions, or symbols, and it doesn't necessarily require visualisation either, because while you might choose to imagine that there are hands treating those areas, you can just as simple allow your attention to rest on those areas and the energy will flow there.

In each position, you merge with the energy and you allow it to flow, to do what it needs to do.

What is different about this meditation, though, is your attention: you direct the flow of energy by focus your attention on a particular area. This is a powerful thing to do because where you focus your attention is where the energy focuses itself.

By allowing your attention to rest on the areas of need, you intensify and boost the flow of energy because "where thought goes, energy flows".

And you can just be there as a bystander in the process, observing, experiencing, in a neutral way: merged with the energy and following the flow of energy.

Over to you

If this self-treatment method is new to you, why not give it a try?

Intuitive hands-on self-treatment method

In previous articles I have been talking about meditative approaches to self-treatment, where you either:

- Meditate with the intention to heal... and just let it happen
- Follow the flow of energy and focus your attention on where the energy is focusing itself
- Direct the flow of energy by resting your attention on different areas of the body

Now I'm going to turn my attention to hands-on self-treatments, but with a bit of a twist. Out go standard self-treatment hand-positions and in comes...

Taggart's Intuitive hands-on self-treatment method

- Make yourself comfortable in a seated or supine position, maybe with your hands folded over each other in front of your chest
- Close your eyes
- Start to become aware of your connection to the energy, your connection to Reiki
- Notice how that connection feels, with the energy engulfing you and building within you in just the right way for you in this moment
- As the energy flows, just remind yourself that your intention now is to heal, to heal on all levels, to rejuvenate, to rebalance

- Just say to yourself, "this is my time to heal now"
- And allow the energy to flow, to flow to wherever it needs to go to give you just what you need in this moment
- *And start to become aware of the energy and where it's flowing*
- *Where is the Reiki focusing itself, where is it dwelling?*
- *Move your hands to rest on, or near, that area*
- *Allow your hands to drift to the best place for them to be*
- *Stay in that position for as long as you need to*
- *If the energy moves on to another area, if your hands want to move on to another area, let that happen*
- *Allow the energy to guide you*
- And finally bring yourself back when you feel ready, and open your eyes

Although this method involves resting your hands on your body – whereas in all the previous self-treatment examples I gave you, you were simply meditating – there are no expectations here.

You rest your hands, and move your hands, according to your individual energy needs during each session.

Each treatment you carry out will most likely be different in some way, as your energy needs vary from one occasion to another.

You might be following the energy, noticing where it wants to flow, and moving your hands to a suitable nearby area.

Or you might find that the hands start to move and drift by themselves, again guided by the energy, giving you exactly what you need on each occasion.

Over to you

If this self-treatment method is new to you, why not give it a try?

The simplest hands-on self-treatment method ever

This is the final article in the series, so I thought I would finish by a very simple hands-on method...

Just rest your hands on yourself and close your eyes

That's it.

That's the method.

Rest your hands on your heart and solar plexus, close your eyes, and let the Reiki flow.

Or rest your hands on your lower abdomen, like in the photo above.

Bliss out on the energy.

Let it go where it wants to go and do what it wants to do.

And when you're done, open your eyes.

Over to you

If this self-treatment method is new to you, why not give it a try?

The "21 Day" thing

Where did the 21 day thing come from?

I wanted to talk a little bit about the "21 day thing": the 21-day self-treat or the 21-day clear-out after attending a First Degree course.

I'm a bit puzzled by this and I've been trying to fathom where it came from, and why it should be recommended.

I think this idea probably came into being because it echoes the story told about Mikao Usui's discovery of Reiki on Mt Kurama where, according to the story that Mrs Takata passed on, Usui Sensei went up Mt Kurama and fasted and meditated for 21 days, culminating in him being hit by a bolt of light, seeing symbols, and Reiki was born.

We know now that this isn't actually what happened: Usui didn't fast for 21 days up the mountain, though he did carry out something called the "Lotus Repentance meditation", and this did last for 21 days I believe.

But this was quite a formalised process – an established Tendai practice – and he went home at night after each day's meditation. In any case, this did not lead to the 'eureka' moment that Mrs Takata spoke about since Usui was already teaching his system before he carried out the first of his Lotus Repentance meditations, and he performed these meditations several times during his lifetime.

7 x 3 = 21

People have speculated and taught that the 21 consecutive days of self-treating is required because the energy makes a visit to each of a person's chakras three times during this period.

The emphasis on chakras within Reiki seems to have originated within Reiki's journey through the New Age movement, where some lineages have incorporated various New Age practices like crystals, spirit guides and Angels etc. Chakra work wasn't part of the original system.

And this three-times-through-your-chakras seems to me to be a bit of 'reverse engineering', where you have something that you're supposed to do, and then you back-track to try and find a justification for it, to make sense of it in your head.

Some suggest that if you carry out a practice for 21 days then you will have established it as a habit, and there may be something in that, actually.

Don't stop after 21 days!

The problem that I have with this idea of a 21-day practice is that some people "do their 21 days" and then stop, or have only a sporadic practice afterwards, as if once you've done your 21 days... that's it, you've cleared yourself out and you don't need to work on yourself so dedicatedly afterwards.

And I also have a problem with the idea that you have a clear-out just during that 21 day period and then you're sorted.

In my experience, the way that people react to Reiki in terms of 'clearing out', whether that be in terms of physical reactions or states of mind or emotions, seems to vary greatly from one person to another. And while Reiki doesn't seem to give people an experience that they can't handle, some can make a great big fast clear-out initially, some have it happening in dribs and drabs, while for others the process may be delayed for a while.

Everyone's different. And there's always something more to clear out!

We all live lives, we have stress, we suppress emotions, we fail to deal with things, so if we carry on working with Reiki, there will be stuff that we will need to shift in the future to bring things into balance for us, not just in those first few weeks.

And just wait until you start attuning people: you may have a mega-clear-out waiting for you!

So while I don't object to people working on themselves dedicatedly for three weeks – why would I? – I'd rather emphasise that if you're going to gain the greatest benefit out of your connection to Reiki then you need to work on yourself regularly.

You don't have to self-treat (or carry out Hatsurei ho) **every** single day (and then beat yourself up for not being perfect if you have to miss a day sometimes) but if you can make Reiki a regular part of your life then you will reap the rewards.

And that's not just for 21 days: that's for life.

Over to you

So, do you have a regular practice of using Reiki on yourself?

And, if so, what have you noticed in terms of the way that your mind/body has responded to that ongoing energy work?

Did you have a bit of a clear-out to begin with, or a great big clear-out, and then occasional ups and downs after then?

Your 10 day Reiki challenge: the "Releasing Exercise"

What is the Releasing Exercise?

I love the way that the Reiki precepts, and the effects of learning Reiki, blend and merge with each other. So if you could encapsulate in words the effects of Reiki on a person, you would probably say that they were largely free from anger and worry and that they were more mindful.

And at the same time we have a set of precepts that encourage us to be mindful, and to let go of worry and anger.

Mikao Usui's precepts are such an important part of the original system and something that can sometimes become overlooked during the head-long rush to get to all the cool energy stuff! But they are really the foundation of Reiki, there to guide us and also to represent and give form to the many changes that Reiki can bring us.

And that got me thinking about whether there was a way of actually using the energy of Reiki to directly experience a precept.

What I came up with was my "Releasing Exercise".

The Releasing Exercise is a way of directly experiencing the effects of a precept in terms of energy flow and the people that I have shared this with have found it to be very powerful.

Maybe you'll find it powerful too.

I am setting you a challenge: to carry out my Releasing Exercise each day for 10 days.

How to perform the Releasing Exercise

I would like to suggest that you do the following, for a couple of minutes at a time, twice a day, for ten days: Sit with your eyes closed and your hands resting in your lap, palms up. You are going to be releasing energy through your hands.

Stage One

Sit comfortably with your eyes closed and your hands resting in your lap, palms up. Take a few long deep breaths and feel yourself becoming peaceful and relaxed. Your mind empties. Say to yourself "I now release all my anger..."; say this three times to yourself if you like. Allow energy to be released through your palms, and be still until the flow of energy subsides. This may take a little while, particularly the first time you try this exercise.

Stage Two

Now say to yourself "I now release all my worry..."; say this three times to yourself if you like. Again allow a flurry of energy to leave your hands and be still until it subsides. Again this may take a little while, particularly the first time you try this exercise.

Try this variation

I really like this variation: try carrying out the releasing exercise in time with your breath. Breathe in gently, say to yourself "I now release all my anger..." and then breathe out, allowing your anger to flood out of you on the out breath, flooding out of your palms. Gently breathe in, and repeat.

Let Taggart Talk You Through It

If you'd like me to talk you through the exercise, go to the Reiki Evolution blog and search for 'releasing exercise'. You'll find an audio track there.

Here's what people experienced

I have included some representative feedback below, so you can see the sort of thing that the exercise has done for people.

Here's what I received from Loretta in Iowa, who has started to use the exercise with her clients:

"I use the release in the morning as I lay in Relaxation pose after finishing yoga and when I feel an emotion I need to work with during the day. I use it for more than anger and worries and the feeling leaving my hands is very emotional. I have also begun using in it in my Reiki practice. I take my clients through breathing exercises and relaxation steps and depending on what is going on with them I introduce the releasing exercise either before the Reiki session or at the end of the session.

Practicing the release is so healing on many levels, it allows us to focus on one issue at a time, allows us to take time for ourself, to dig deep on issues we may want to push to the background. This process makes my day wonderful, I feel so much more on an even keel with the world and with myself."

Emma in Scotland has experimented with the exercise, focusing the energy on releasing other emotions:

"I have tried the 10 day releasing exercise and found it really beneficial – I'm going to continue doing it everyday. It's really effective and so simple! I have a lot of bottled up emotion and I feel much more relaxed after doing this and feel quite a powerful flow of energy leaving my body.

I have tried other variations which also seem to work such as saying "I release sadness" or "regret" or sometimes even "I release any unnecessary or unhelpful emotion". I even tried it lying down imagining the energy flowing out through the soles of my feet so that I could do it last thing at night before going to sleep. I'm not sure that's as effective but I did feel relaxed! Anyway, thank you for the idea and I will continue to use it."

Here's what I received from Vivien in the UK, who found the exercise worked well when dealing with a difficult issue that arose:

"Well your exercises arrived at a very good time for me. We had a very difficult "political/social" issue at work whereby I got so angry (on someone else's behalf). This person had offloaded her problems to me and I was surprised how angry I felt inside at the injustice that she had suffered. It was one of those situations I took home with me.

I did offer her advice and suggested various courses of action which helped her but, despite that, I still had this real burning anger inside me which I took home with me on a Friday. I did your 'anger releasing'exercises on the Friday and over the weekend and it certainly helped! I practiced it a few times each day and hey presto, I was chilled by the Monday and everything has now been resolved thankfully!

I didn't need to do it for 10 days but in future if I find myself in a similar situation, I will know what to do. I will also try out the others. So a big thank you!!!!"

Teresa in the UK sent me her feedback, and she found that the exercise helped her to just 'be':

"This is a wonderful exercise for letting go of anger and worry. The more I practised this the more I became lighter and freer in my thoughts and actions. Being in the present, no past, no future, simply alive in the moment.

Thank you very much for this."

Paul from the UK contacted me to say that the exercise helped to change his perception of things:

"I'm very new to Reiki and started your releasing exercise as another "string to my bow". Before starting my Reiki journey, I was already practicing mindful meditation. I've found your release exercise a natural extension of this.

I work in a quite highly stressed office environment, a place where small irritations can rapidly grow into something more. I'm generally very relaxed and laid back anyway, but over the last ten days my colleagues have seen fit to comment about how even MORE laid back I seem to have become.

I've been self-reflecting on this. At first I thought the exercise was helping me become more tolerant, but I now realise that's not the case at all. "Tolerance" is more about "putting up with the irritation". I think I would say I now have more "acceptance". Because I'm free from anger and worry, I can "accept" things that would have been seen as irritants. Because I "accept" them, I don't have to "tolerate" them.

I've passed your exercise to a number of my Reiki friends who expressed an interest. I'm waiting to hear back from them."

Pat explained how the exercise has helped her with two specific situations recently:

"I started the releasing exercise before Chistmas and have found it very effective. I felt the release of energy in my palms and very often in my third eye area. I sometimes felt warmth, almost like a hot flush!!!

Two things happened during the time that I was doing the exercise which would have normally been very upsetting under normal circumstances but I dealt with it using this practice. I have tried both ways of the practice as you suggested and they were both equally effective.

The first situation that I mentioned above was a very cutting comment made by someone which was hurtful and as soon as it happened, I did the release exercise and the effect was very comforting. The second was some health news that made me angry and concerned. I again used the practice to release the anger, worry and blame. I found the exercise very helpful in both of those situations.

I have continued to do the practice and yesterday started to add fear as well as anger and worry to my routine. I will definitely continue with this exercise. I am very grateful to you and thank you very much for telling us about this."

Finally, Marilynne explains how she feels that this exercise is very much in line with the way that we do things at Reiki Evolution:

"I have not done the releasing exercise regularly over 10 days. However when I do use it, it is very effective in releasing thoughts of both worry and anger, the two detrimental, mischievous little devils that can be so disruptive in their negativity. I cherish the precepts and accept them as powerful ideals and daily reminders. I have just had my Reiki 2 session last weekend and feel the energy so much stronger now through my hand and down to the tan-den. The releasing exercise seems so natural, and very much 'in tune' with all that I have learned and experienced through Reiki Evolution. Practicing control of the flow of Reiki energy, including the release of worry and anger, is just a wonderful privilege."

Time For You To Take The 10 Day Releasing Exercise Challenge!

So now it's over to you: your turn to carry out my releasing exercise for ten days, if you want to!

Using Reiki for anxiety

Does Reiki work for Anxiety?

I think a lot of people come to Reiki wondering if it can help ease their anxiety, and I think that there is a general sense that Reiki can help you to become more calm and chilled. So is Reiki good for anxiety? Will it help you to let go of those worries?

Well in my experience, yes, Reiki does really work to help reduce anxiety and there are three ways that it does this, I think.

1. Through mindfulness
2. Through the use of the Reiki precepts
3. Through meditating on and using the Reiki energy

What is Anxiety?

When we worry, we are thinking about the future and what might happen to us or the people we care about. We imagine a frightening or unhappy future and that makes us scared.

And since we have fairly prehistoric brains and responses, we respond to this future threat like it was some sort of sabre-toothed tiger in front of us: we go into 'flight, fright or freeze' mode, with elevated heart rate, high blood pressure and the like.

Long term, this is not good for our bodies since our immune system is dampened down and blood is rerouted away from our digestive systems, so we end up run down, prone to infection and with digestive disturbances.

All because we are responding to an imaginary future.

How can Reiki help Anxiety?

There are two important aspects of Reiki training that work together to ease anxiety: mindfulness and the Reiki precepts I'm not going to go into detail about these in this article, since I have spoken about them elsewhere, but these two aspects of Reiki training very much work with each other to reduce anxiety.

The Reiki precepts start with the phrase "just for today" and that emphasises the idea of mindfulness, where you are fully immersed in the moment, fully engaged with what you are doing. "Just for today" exhorts us, just for this moment, to be content, to be compassionate and forgiving of ourselves, to be aware of the many blessings that we have in our lives.

If you are mindful then there are no thoughts about the past or the future: you are embracing the present moment, and when you do this it's not easy to worry (because you can only do this when you send yourself off into an imagined negative future).

Although mindfulness isn't emphasised or even mentioned on a lot of Reiki courses, it is an important part of the original system that Mikao Usui taught and is something that we explain and encourage as soon as you start your Reiki training with us.

Reiki energy and Anxiety

But beyond the practice of mindfulness, and the benefits that come when introducing the Reiki principles into your daily life, there is something else going on too. because when you are 'connected' to Reiki, when you are aware of and working with the energy through daily energy exercises and meditations, changes take place within you that very much echo the benefits of mindfulness and precepts-work.

Reiki, in itself – Reiki, the energy – helps people to feel more calm, content and serene, better able to cope with difficult situations and people. Working with Reiki helps you to come back into contact with that core part of you that is balanced and centred, a still foundation that can weather the storms that life often throws at us.

Do you already have Reiki?

If so, and if you feel that there is still a bit more work to be done in terms of leaving worry behind, there are a couple of techniques I created that I think will be of great help to you. You can read about them in other articles. Here are the titles:

- Releasing exercise
- Precepts rehearsal

These exercises allow you to use the Reiki energy as a 'carrier' to disperse or dissipate any accumulated worry, and also help you to set a new course, so you respond differently in the future. These exercises are deceptively powerful and should be carried out for several weeks to gain the full benefit from them.

Using Reiki for stress

Can Reiki help with Stress?

In my last article I was talking about how Reiki can help with Anxiety and while stress and anxiety are often lumped together as if they were the same things, there is quite a difference between these two experiences in terms of what's going on.

Where anxiety is a fear of an imagined future, where you feel frightened about things that are yet to happen and may not actually happen, with stress you are reflecting on how you believe you're going to be able to cope with different tasks or events. Stress is all about "I can't do this", "I'm not going to be able to do this".

So stress is all about how competent you believe you are and becoming frightened about letting yourself down, or letting other people down. Stress is about losing face, not succeeding in a particular task or goal, it's about fear of showing that you're not good enough.

Using Reiki for Stress relief

So **can Reiki help with stress** and, if so, how does that happen?

Well, I think it comes down to the three powerful aspects of the Reiki that we introduce to students on our First Degree courses: mindfulness, the Reiki precepts and regular energy work.

I'm not going to go into a lot of detail about mindfulness because I have written about it before, but when you are mindful you are fully engaged in and engrossed with the task at hand, whether that doing the washing up or going for a walk. You become fully aware of the experience of you doing the task, living fully in the present moment, with no thoughts of the future or the past.

You might notice the flow of energy through your nostrils, the feeling in the soles of your feet as you walk, the sounds of birdsong, the myriad of colours that are before you, the sensation of soap suds on your fingertips, the swishing of the water. You notice your thoughts pass by like clouds.

In doing so you start to come into contact with a still, calm centre that we all have within us if we give ourselves a chance to experience it, that place from which we can observe, non-judgmentally.

It is in this still place where we can let go of those feelings of stress, setting us free, and the more we practise mindfulness, the more often and more easily can we ease into that helpful state.

The Reiki precepts and stress

The Reiki precepts (or the Reiki principles, or 'Gokai') are a simple set of 'rules to live by' that were established and taught by Reiki's founder, Mikao Usui. There were said to distil the essence of Tendai Buddhist teachings into a simple set of guiding principles that anyone can follow.

The Reiki precepts emphasise humility and compassion: compassion for ourselves as much as compassion for others.

So how can we be compassionate towards ourselves and how can that help with stress?

Well, we can forgive ourselves, we can give ourselves a break and forgive ourselves for not being perfect. If we expect ourselves to be perfect then no matter how hard we work, no matter how much we achieve, no matter what we do or try to do, we will never be happy.

So we can give ourselves some self-love and understanding, we can nurture ourselves, and the best place from which to do this is from that still, calm centre that we gain a glimpse of when we are mindful.

Reiki energy and Stress

Tying these strands together – the mindfulness and the compassion and self-forgiveness – is the use of Reiki energy on ourselves.

By having a good, regular routine of working on ourselves using Reiki – by carrying out daily energy exercises and some form of self-treatment – we nudge our energy system more into a state of balance, bathing us in calm, helping us to fully experience that content, still core, and putting us in the best possible position to really benefit from this wonderful system.

Oh, and I just wanted to mention that although in this article I am talking about learning Reiki as a way of managing your stress, receiving Reiki treatments on a regular basis is also a wonderful way of experiencing the powerful balancing effect of this simple hands-on therapy.

Can you send distant healing at Reiki first degree?

An unnecessary piece of dogma

It is taught commonly on Reiki courses that you aren't able to do distant healing at First Degree and that you can only send distant healing once you've been 'attuned' to the distant healing symbol.

I don't agree with that and think it's unnecessarily dogmatic and limiting… and makes no sense!

Firstly, distant healing isn't something that is unique to Reiki: many spiritual healers practise this. So we have a group of people who haven't been attuned to Reiki at all, they haven't been 'attuned' to anything in a Reiki sense, and they can send distant healing.

So are we saying that people who haven't been attuned to Reiki are able to send distant healing, but once you're attuned to First Degree then this ability somehow stops, only to start again when you've been on a Second Degree course?

That makes no sense!

And let's think about the Buddhist origins of Reiki: one of the principles of Buddhism is that reality is illusion, the idea of us being separate individuals, distinct from other people, is illusion, and that the true reality is that of oneness.

Mikao Usui was a Buddhist.

Mainly, he taught people who were Buddhists or followers of Shinto.

Would he have established an energetic system, when his whole worldview was based on the idea of oneness, that suddenly went against this grain and introduced the idea that people at First Degree were in some way exempt from this basic Buddhist principle of oneness?

I don't think so.

Distant Healing at First Degree

So we teach the basics of distant healing on our First Degree course, and why wouldn't we, since it's an essential part of the energy system that we use. We teach a simple approach, but it doesn't need to be complicated.

We don't teach the 'distant healing symbol' (referred to as 'HSZSN') on First Degree and we don't need to because you don't need to use that symbol, or be 'attuned' to it, in order to send distant healing effectively.

When we do teach the distant healing symbol on Second Degree, certainly it does provide a useful focus, though to be honest I prefer to use the corresponding kotodama instead since I believe that this mantra helps to make connections on a whole new level, whether working on someone in person or at a distance.

Experiment

If you're currently at First Degree, why not experiment with distant healing and see what's possible.

To get you started if you're not sure what to do, take a look at the article called "The simplest distant healing method ever!": anyone can use it; it's symbol free and it works well.

At Reiki Evolution we're happy for our students to experiment and find their own way with the energy: we don't want out students to turn into clones of us!

Restrictions on Reiki

Depending on whom you trained with, you may have been given quite a long list of 'situations where you should not use Reiki'. It seems that the only restriction that Mrs Takata taught was that you should not treat a broken bone with Reiki, but many other restrictions have been added in later on in Reiki's Western history. I thought I would spend a little time talking about these 'Reiki contraindications'.

The "broken bone" thing

Firstly, I would like to talk about the 'broken bone' restriction. This is made on the basis that Reiki accelerates the healing process, so you do not want Reiki to set the bone before it has been put back in the right position.

Now while Reiki is an amazing energy, and has done some wonderful and breathtaking things, I think most people's experience is that Reiki gently supports the body's natural healing ability, and that while it may accelerate the healing process, the effects of Reiki generally build up cumulatively. I do not believe that Reiki will set someone's bone like fast-acting Polyfilla, so that they will have to have the bone re-broken and re-set when they get to Casualty a few hours later.

Breaking a bone is a shocking and painful experience (I know this from first hand experience!) and Reiki could make a real difference to someone, so I would not hold back from giving it, and I would not hold back from treating the area where the bone is broken.

Suggesting that you could Reiki someone, but keep well away from the broken bone, does not stop Reiki from rushing to where it is needed (the bone), and why would we imagine that what many people see as a spiritually-guided life-force energy would mess things up for a person. Reiki is supposed to be intelligent.

Reiki and pacemakers

Another situation where some people are taught that you 'should not treat' is when a client has a pacemaker. This restriction is made on the basis that Reiki energy is electromagnetic in nature, and will interfere with the proper functioning of the device.

Confusingly, some say that this restriction only applies to analogue pacemakers, not the newer digital ones.

There seems to be no evidence whatsoever to indicate that Reiki would cause a problem in this area, and I have not heard on a single anecdote where a Reiki practitioner treated someone with a pacemaker and the treatment caused problems.

I am also not aware of any evidence to show that Reiki is electromagnetic in nature, either. If it was, you could measure Reiki easily: move your hand over a wire and you would induce an electric current, which you could pick up with a voltmeter.

Some have suggested that you can solve this 'problem' by keeping away from the heart area, but we all know that Reiki rushes from where we put it to where it is needed.

I would have thought that a person with a pacemaker needed more Reiki in the heart area, not less, and if Reiki is drawn to the areas of need then it is going to go where it wants anyway. The only solution would be not to treat someone with a pacemaker, which I think is ridiculous.

Some have suggested that you should not attune someone with a pacemaker, and again I do not think that this is sensible. I am not going to restrict my practice of Reiki on the basis of unfounded supposition.

Where is the evidence?

With nearly all the restrictions that are put on Reiki, there seems to be no evidence to back up any of them. I am not talking about double blind clinical trials here, but even simple anecdotes where a practitioner has treated someone and found that there is a problem that can be reasonably attributed to the treatment that has been given.

I have heard that you should not treat insulin-dependent Diabetics, or people taking steroids for adrenal insufficiency. Those restrictions have been made on the basis that if Reiki produces an instant cure then the patient's next dose of insulin, or steroids, will kill them.

Again, while Reiki is a wonderful healing force, it is not my belief that Reiki is likely to cure diabetes, for example, at the click of a finger.

Most people's experience is that the effects of Reiki build up cumulatively and that if a condition has taken a long time to develop, then it is not so likely to disappear straight away. Yes, a diabetic patient's blood glucose levels may vary after a Reiki treatment, but diabetics' blood sugar levels vary a great deal anyway. That is why they have to keep on sticking themselves with a pin to monitor their levels, and you could only attribute this variation to Reiki if it happened consistently after treatments and their blood sugar levels were stable the rest of the time.

Having said that, there does seem to be some anecdotal evidence that Reiki treatments can sometimes cause the client's blood sugar levels to alter after a treatment. This does not mean that you should not treat diabetics: it means that you need to keep this in mind and mention this possibility to the client, so that they can monitor their blood sugar levels accordingly.

Waking up and falling asleep

I have heard that you should not send distant Reiki to someone who is driving a car, because they will fall asleep, and you should not send distant Reiki to someone who is under an anaesthetic, because it will make them wake up... well, which is it? This doesn't sound like an intelligent energy to me, and there seems to be a lot of fear, and a lack of trust in the energy, underlying all these restrictions.

So where is the evidence that Reiki wakes people up during surgery? Where is even one anecdote where it was clear that Reiki, rather than any other cause, led to this happening?

Look for the evidence, and you find that these scare stories have no foundation.

Cancer, pregnancy, depression, asthma, stress, homoeopathy, animals, medicines

In fact, the restrictions do not stop there. There are many more taught in different lineages. For example, you should not treat people with cancer, you should not treat people who are pregnant, you should not treat people who are depressed or who have asthma, you should not treat people who are stressed, you should not treat young children, you should not treat animals, you should not treat people who are taking homoeopathic remedies, you should not treat people who are taking medicines, you should not treat people wearing green trousers (sorry, I made that one up!).

Let's just examine two of these. It is said by some teachers that you should not treat people who have cancer because Reiki will "feed the cancer"; there is a variation on this myth, actually, where people are taught that they should not use one of the Reiki symbols because it will "put energy into the cancer".

Let's think rationally about this for just a second: we have cancer cells inside us all of the time and as you sit reading this, there are cancer cells in you. Your cells go haywire all the time and your immune system detects the errors and kills the cells. But if you adhere to this Reiki contraindication then you should not treat anyone at all because Reiki feeds cancer cells, and everyone has cancer cells in them, so we can't treat people, or animals, we can't treat ourselves, and being attuned would be a death sentence!

And if we can't treat pregnant women then we really need to refrain from treating any women of childbearing age because of course women can be in the early stages of pregnancy and not know about it, or be pregnant and not know about it. And then of course all women of childbearing age should refrain from self-treating, and should not go on Reiki courses.

People do not think things through.

I believe that Reiki is a beautiful healing energy that supports the body's natural healing ability, and brings things into balance on all levels. It either has an innate intelligence, and knows where to go to an extent, or it is the body that is intelligent and draws the energy to where it is needed.

In either case, Reiki is not going to mess up a person and leave them less well off than they were before they started, other than a temporary intensification of symptoms.

Examples of these would be an emotional release or strong emotions felt for a few days after being treated, or joint pains getting worse during a treatment and then improving subsequently.

Distant healing

The last set of restrictions that I have heard about concern distant healing, where it is said in some quarters that you should not send Reiki to people who have not asked for or given their permission.

Some people say that it is totally unethical to send distant Reiki to someone without obtaining their agreement and that it a gross intrusion. I do not agree with this, for a number of reasons:

1. Firstly, I see sending distant Reiki as rather like sending concentrated prayer. When you pray for someone you are asking for Divine intervention in another person's life, in whatever way is right for that person according to Divine will. You are asking for things to change for the better. When you send Reiki you are sending it with loving intent and for the person's highest good, so it is in line with that person's destiny or karma, and many people see Reiki energy as having Divine origins. You do not ring someone up to ask their permission to pray for them, so why should if be different with Reiki?

2. If someone were knocked over by a car a few yards away from you, would you really not send Reiki to them because you couldn't drag them into the seated position to sign a consent form? No. You would send Reiki to their highest good and let the energy do what is appropriate for them. You offer the energy: you do not force the recipient to receive it.

3. Reiki is a beautiful healing energy that brings things into balance on all levels and does not mess people up, leaving them worse off than they were to begin with. With distant healing your intent is that the energy works for the highest good of the recipient, so if it is not appropriate for that person to get the benefit of the energy then it simply will not work. You are not imposing your will and you are not imposing your preferred solution on the situation. You are simply sending love, offering the energy, making the energy available, not forcing it to be received.

For these reasons, I have no problem in sending Reiki to people who have not specifically requested it. I send the energy with the intention that it be received by the recipient at whatever time is appropriate for them.

I do not see that there are any other restrictions that need to be applied to the energy, or the practice of Reiki.

In the West we think too much, and come up with too many complications. Reiki is simple and does not need to be restricted.

It knows what to do.

Intelligent Energy?

It is well established within Reiki that the energy we channel is 'intelligent'. Some people believe that the energy is innately intelligent, perhaps because of its divine origins, and some believe that the intelligence of the energy is accounted for by the presence of spirit guides who direct the energy as we treat someone.

Others believe that it is the body that is intelligent, drawing the energy to where it needs to go.

Most of us will have noticed that the energy will move from where our hands are resting to other parts of the recipient's body, drawn according to the recipient's need to areas of need, so it is clear that it doesn't always restrict itself to where we place it.

Some people take the line that Reiki will work perfectly well no matter what hand positions you use, irrespective of the knowledge and experience of the practitioner and whether or not the practitioner can work intuitively.

The implication of this is that you could quite happily carry out a Reiki treatment by simply holding someone's hands for an hour and the energy would be drawn to the areas of need, and that there is nothing that you could do to help make the treatment more effective.

Another view is that there are things that a practitioner can do in order to increase the effectiveness of a treatment, for example:

- Working on yourself to develop your ability as a channel
- Using intuition to decide where to put your hands (rather than following standard hand positions) and what aspect of the energy to emphasise during the treatment, or where to direct your attention.

There are some inconsistencies in the first view described above. Many people will use techniques designed to balance the chakras, while at the same time maintaining that Reiki is intelligent and will always give the recipient what they need. Yet imposing your will on the energy and using it to balance the chakras is over-riding the way that the energy will work in the body, is it not?

Surely if Reiki is an intelligent energy then it will balance the recipient's chakras in a way that is appropriate for the individual, without the practitioner doing anything specific to achieve this.

If you routinely direct Reiki to balance a person's chakras you are suggesting that Reiki will not balance the chakras without direct intervention by the practitioner. Since most people would agree that Reiki works on your energy system and produces beneficial effects on all levels, how could it not balance your chakras during this process?

Either Reiki is intelligent, in which case you don't need to spend time balancing people's chakras, or it isn't intelligent, in which case we would always need to move in to balance the chakras.

But if Reiki can't even balance your chakras on its own, what on earth is it doing?

I believe that spending time balancing people's chakras using Reiki is unnecessary, and that Reiki will do to a person's chakras what needs to be done to achieve balance for them at the end of a treatment.

Of course subsequently the chakras will drift out of balance again, back to their more habitual state, but I believe that by repeating a treatment you are showing the chakras what it is like to be in a state of balance, and that repeated exposure to this balanced state, by providing a series of treatments, helps to move the recipient's chakras more into a state of balance long-term.

Another challenge to the 'Reiki is perfectly intelligent, we do not need to develop ourselves as a channel, we do not need to work intuitively" point of view is the fact that people are able to develop an intuitive ability and find that their hands are guided into combinations of hand positions that are different from one person to another, and different from one treatment to another.

This suggests, of course, that there are sequences of hand positions that are more appropriate or effective in dealing with an individual's problems on that occasion than simply applying a standard template.

If a standard template is always sufficient – or just holding someone's hands for an hour is all that is needed – why would our hands be guided by the energy to direct the energy into particular areas, distinctive for that recipient and different from the hand positions elicited for another person?

Intuitive working

In practice, I have found that people treated with intuitively-guided hand positions find that the energy seems to penetrate more deeply, that the treatments feel in some way more relevant, more profound, more effective than when standard positions are used, and that is my impression too.

Treatments based on intuitively-guided hand positions seem more powerful, sometimes a lot more powerful, than treatments based on standard hand positions, since we are directing the energy into just the right combination, and sequence, of positions for that person on that occasion.

If we look to the origins of Reiki and the way that Mikao Usui taught, we can see that intuitive working was a fundamental part of the practice of Reiki, and still is in Mikao Usui's Reiki Association in Japan to this day.

Why would Usui have placed so much emphasis on using intuition if standard hand positions - or no hand positions - are just as good in terms of producing good results? He was a practical man, after all. So there is something special about working intuitively: it seems to do more than standard hand positions can.

Hand positions for different ailments

For the benefit of students who could not yet work intuitively (and that is the important point), Chujiro Hayashi produced a long list of what could be described as 'good places to put your hands for different medical conditions', which suggests that certain combinations of hand positions are more effective in dealing with specific conditions that applying a standard template.

Why would Dr Hayashi have produced such a list if, as many believe, Reiki is an intelligent energy that always goes where it is needed? We should remember, though, that this list was a stopgap, and that intuitive working was the ideal.

The above suggests that although Reiki may be intelligent to an extent – or the recipient's body is intelligent to an extent – we can enhance our treatments through some of the things that we can do, for example allowing the energy to guide us in terms of where we place our hands.

Further inconsistencies in the 'Reiki is perfectly intelligent' point of view come through the use of symbols: if we think about it, as soon as we start using any of the Reiki symbols in the Western fashion, perhaps routinely drawing the symbols as we treat, in a pre-determined sequence, we are consciously over-riding the way that the energy wants to work when left to its own devices, and imposing our will by directing the energy in a certain way.

Yet if the energy knows exactly what to and where to go, why would we need to use symbols? Why would we need to impose our control over the energy in this way?

But this is not the only way that the symbols can be used. Just in the same way that we can move beyond standard hand positions to embrace intuitive working, with all the benefits that are associated with this, we can also work intuitively when we use the symbols, allowing the energy to guide us in terms of which aspect of the energy we emphasise, if any, during a treatment. Thus we work in partnership with the energy.

I believe that Reiki is an intelligent energy to an extent, and is drawn by the recipient's need to the appropriate areas, sometimes over-riding the way that we have directed the energy if that is required.

However, we can assist in providing just what the recipient needs on each occasion by working intuitively, by being open and allowing the energy to guide us.

I believe that we work in partnership with the energy, and that we are not simply empty tubes through which the energy flows.

Through the development of our intuition, we can understand how the energy needs to be directed by us to better help our clients: where best to put our hands, and what aspects of the energy need to be emphasised.

Developing your Reiki

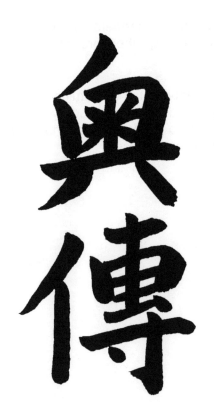

Back to Basics: Reiki Second Degree

People learn Reiki for many reasons and come from an amazing variety of backgrounds, all attending for their own personal reasons. Reiki courses in the UK present a whole variety of approaches, some "traditional" Western-style, some more Japanese in content, some wildly different and almost unrecognisable, some free and intuitive, others dogmatic and based on rules about what you should always do and not do. Reiki is taught in so many ways, and students will tend to imagine that the way that they were taught is the way that Reiki is taught and practised by most other Reiki people.

What I have tried to do in this article is to present a simple guide to what in my view is the essence of Second Degree: what it's all about and what we should be doing and thinking about to get the most out of our experience of Reiki at this level.

My words are addressed to anyone at Second Degree level, or anyone who would like to review the essence of Second Degree.

The first thing I want to say is that there should usually be an interval of a couple of months or so between First and Second Degree if you want to get the most out of your Reiki experience, and that it is unwise to take both Degrees back-to-back over a weekend. We would not take an advanced driving test the day after passing our basic driving test, so why would we believe that moving on to a more 'advanced' level with Reiki would be an effective way to learn when we have had no opportunity to get the hang of the basics of First Degree?

Can we get the most out of Second Degree when we have had no opportunity to get used to working with and sensing and experiencing energy, when we have had no opportunity to enhance our effectiveness as a channel and our sensitivity to Reiki through regular practice, when we have had no opportunity to become familiar with a standard treatment routine and have had no opportunity to feel comfortable and confident in treating other people?

Reiki is not a race, and we need to be familiar with the basics before moving on.

Second Degree is all about:

1. reinforcing or enhancing your connection to the energy
2. learning some symbols which you can use routinely when working on yourself or treating others
3. enhancing your self-healing
4. learning how to effect a strong distant connection (distant healing)

And ideally it is also about opening yourself up to your intuitive side so that you throw away the basic Reiki 'rule book' and go freestyle, gearing any treatments towards the individual needs of the recipient.

There are many approaches to doing these things, and I wanted below to touch on each one and to dispel some myths that may have been passed on.

Enhancing your Connection to the energy

On your Second Degree course you will have received some attunements or some empowerments. Attunements are not standard rituals within the world of Reiki and take many forms, some simpler and some more complex. They have evolved and changed greatly during their journey from teacher to teacher in the West.

There is no "right way" to carry out an attunement and the individual details of a ritual do not matter a great deal. They all work. Equally, there is no "correct" number of attunements that have to be carried out at Second Degree level. Whether you receive one, two, or three attunements on your course, that is fine.

On your course you may have received some "empowerments" rather than attunements, though these are less common. The word "empowerment", or "Reiju empowerment", refers to a connection ritual that has come to us from some Japanese sources, and is closer in essence to the empowerment that Mikao Usui conveyed to his students. If you are receiving empowerments rather than attunements then you really need to have received three of them at least.

What we experience when receiving an attunement or an empowerment will vary a lot. Some people have fireworks and bells and whistles and that's nice for them; other people notice a lot less, or very little, or even nothing, and that's fine too. What we feel when we have an attunement is not a guide to how well it has worked for us. Attunements work, and sometimes we will have a strong experience, but it's not compulsory!

Whether we have noticed a lot, or very little, the attunement will have given us what we need.

Since in Mikao Usui's system you would have received empowerments from him again and again, it would be nice if you could echo this practice by receiving further empowerments (or attunements) and perhaps these might be available at your teacher's Reiki shares or get-togethers, if they hold them. But it is possible to receive distant Reiju empowerments and various teachers make them freely available as a regular 'broadcast'.

This is not essential, and your connection to Reiki once given does not fizzle out, but it would be a beneficial practice if you could receive regular empowerments from someone.

Being "attuned" to a symbol

For many years within the world of Reiki, people believed that the symbols would not work for you, that they were essentially useless, until you had been "attuned" to the symbol: then it would work for you. Unfortunately the only connection rituals available in the West were 'attunements' which involved attuning you to a symbol, so no-one knew how to carry out a 'symbol-free' attunement to see if you really needed to be attuned to a symbol for it to work for you.

But in 1999, from Japan, emerged Reiju empowerments, a representation of the empowerments that Usui conferred, and these empowerments do not use symbols. Finally we were able to see if you really needed to be attuned to a symbol for it to work for you. Lo and behold we discovered that the symbols work fine for people who are connected to the energy using Reiju; they work fine for people who are connected to Reiki but who have not been 'attuned' to the symbols. It seems that once you are connected to Reiki – and now we know how to achieve this without symbols entering into the process – the symbols will work for you, and in fact any symbol seems to push the energy in a particular direction without you having to be specifically 'attuned' to it (whatever that means).

The Reiki symbols are simply graphical representations of different aspects of the energy, a way of representing and emphasising what is already there.

"Sacred Symbols"

In some lineages students are not allowed to keep copies of the symbols and have to reproduce them from memory, based on what they learned on their Second Degree course.

There is the suggestion that the symbols are sacred and not only sacred but secret, and should not be shown to people who are not involved in Reiki, or people who are at First Degree level. Where this idea came from in the Western Reiki system is not clear, since certainly Dr Hayashi had his students copy out his notes by way of preparing their own manuals, including copying down the symbols.

For me, the Reiki symbols are simply graphical representations of different aspects of the energy, useful tools to assist us in experiencing or becoming consciously aware of different aspects of what we already have, and what is special or sacred is our connection to the source, not the squiggles we might put on a piece of paper.

Because of the 'Chinese whispers' that have resulted from students not being allowed to take home hard copies of the Reiki symbols, there are many different versions of the symbols in existence, but they are mainly variations on a theme and they all seem to work in practice.

Do remember, though, that the original CKR had an anticlockwise spiral, and to use a version of CKR with a clockwise spiral is to use a symbol that is not part of the Usui/Hayashi/Takata system.

Using Symbols in practice

Some students are taught there is one 'correct' way that symbols have to be used. Reiki is not so finicky. The important thing when using a Reiki symbol is to focus your attention on the symbol in some way, so whether you are drawing the symbol with your fingers hovering over the back of your hand as you treat someone, whether you are drawing out the symbol using eye movements, or nose movements, or in your mind's eye, all approaches will work.

You do not need to visualise the symbols in a particular colour and if you can see the symbol in your mind's eye in its entirety – this takes practice - you can 'flash' the whole symbol rather than drawing it out stroke by stroke.

Just because we have been taught some symbols does not mean that we are now obliged to use them all the time when we treat or when we work on ourselves. They can be used to emphasise different aspects of the energy, but this is optional. Use of symbols does seem to boost the flow of energy, so we can use them when it feels appropriate.

This is the key: to bring a symbol into a particular part of a treatment when we have a strong feeling that we ought to, to work intuitively rather than following a set method.

I have written in other articles about the issue of simplicity within Reiki practice, and the complicated way that people have ended up using the Reiki symbols, for example mixing symbols together or using complicated symbol sandwiches. Remember that the simple approach is usually the most effective, and that there is no hard and fast way that you 'have' to work with the symbols you have been shown.

By the way, if you have been taught that you have to draw the three Second Degree symbols over your palm each day or else they will stop working for you, you can safely ignore these instructions. The symbols will work for you no matter what you do or don't do with your palms!

Why the symbols are there

At Second Degree, the prime focus of Reiki is still your self-healing, and the first two symbols are there to help you get to grips with two important energies that will further or deepen your self-healing. Putting the 'distant healing' symbol to one side, the other two symbols represent the energies of earth ki and heavenly ki, and we need to fully assimilate these two energies to enhance our self-healing and self-development. If we are going to use these energies when we treat other people, it makes sense to be thoroughly familiar with these energies, to have spent time 'becoming' these energies. We can do this by carrying out regular symbol meditations.

Making 'distant' connections

The third Reiki symbol that you are introduced to on a Second Degree course is commonly called the 'distant healing symbol'.

We should remember that distant healing is perfectly possible at First Degree level and that we do not need to use a symbol in order to send Reiki to another person: intent is enough. But using this symbol can help us to learn to better 'click' into a nice strong merged state.

There is no set form of ritual that 'has' to be used in distant healing, there is not set form of words that has to be recited, no established sequence which needs to be reproduced in order for distant healing to be effective, so we can find our own comfortable approach, different from other people's but equally valid. The details of the ritual that we use are not important.

All we need to do is to focus our attention on the recipient and maybe use the symbol in some way, merge with the energy, merge with the recipient, and allow the energy to flow.

Intuitive working

Ideally, Second Degree should be the stage where you start to leave the basic 'rulebook' behind and go 'freestyle', gearing your treatment towards the recipient's individual energy needs, so that each treatment will be different, as the recipient's energy needs change from one treatment session to another.

Some students will already be modifying the basic treatment routine by the time that they arrive on their Second Degree course.

Set hand positions and a prescribed scheme to follow are useful things to have at First Degree, and allow the student to feel confident in treating others, but sequences of hand positions can be left behind when we open to intuition. Intuitive treatments seem to do something special for the recipient: when you direct the energy into just the right combination of positions for that person on that occasion you allow the energy to penetrate deeply and this seems to lead to a more profound experience for the recipient.

Treatments using intuitively guided hand positions may involve much fewer hand positions being held, and each combination being held for much longer, than in a 'standard' treatment.

We recommend that the Japanese "Reiji ho" approach is used to help Second Degree students to open to their intuitive side, since the approach is so simple and seems to work for most people even within a few minutes of practice. The resulting strong belief that the student is "intuitive" is a hugely empowering state and opens many doors.

Finally

Reiki has the potential to make an amazing, positive difference to you and the people around you. Remember that Reiki is simplicity itself, and by taking some steps to work on yourself regularly, and share Reiki with the people close to you, you are embarking on a very special journey.

How far you travel on that journey is governed by how many steps you take. Carry on with your Hatsurei and self-treatments, get to grips with the energies of CKR and SHK through regular meditation, find your own comfortable approach to carrying out distant healing, and open yourself to intuitive working.

And have fun!

The Breath of Earth and Heaven

In this article I would like to talk about the energy that we work with when we practise Reiki: when we work on ourselves and when we share Reiki with others. The energy that we channel is described in various ways: we are said to be working with universal energy, we are passing on unconditional love, or chi, or prana. But there are aspects of the energy that are not being explained through this use of words, and in this article I want to talk about the essence of Reiki energy. In doing this we will touch on Taoism, QiGong, Shintoism, meditation, breathing, chanting and the use of the Reiki symbols.

Joshin Kokkyu ho

Now many people reading this article will be practising something called "Joshin Kokkyu Ho", an energy breathing method taught in the Usui Reiki Ryoho Gakkai, the Usui Memorial Society in Japan – part of a longer sequence of exercises referred to as "Hatsurei ho". It was also used in Mikao Usui's original system, according to a group of Usui Sensei's surviving students who are in contact with one or two people in the West.

Joshin Kokkyu Ho translates as something like 'technique for purification of the spirit' or 'soul cleansing breathing method', and on its own 'Kokkyu Ho' means 'the way of breathing'.

When we use this method we are moving energy in time with our breath, into and out of our Tanden (Dantien in Chinese), it is a way of achieving balance, but there is more significance to this technique than simply moving energy through our bodies.

Yin and Yang

With each in-breath we are filling the body with ki. This ki is yin in nature, it is the breath of earth, of physicality and the power of separation. By contrast the out-breath distributes ki throughout our bodies. This is yang in nature, it is the breath of heaven, of spirituality and the power of unification. So from the moment that we practise Joshin Kokkyu Ho we are experiencing earth ki and heavenly ki.

In fact, earth ki and heavenly ki are what we are: we are physical reality and we are spiritual essence.

In Taoist philosophy, Earth and Heaven – along with Humanity – are known as the "Three Powers". Humanity is in a pivotal position between the cosmic powers of heaven and the natural forces of earth, covered by heaven above and supported by earth below.

Qi Gong, the energy cultivation technique which is practised in Japan as 'kiko', allows us to work with these two energies and bring them into balance. Shinto practices also refer to these two basic energies, these two essential aspects of what we really are.

It is not surprising, then, that these two energies are the basis of Usui Sensei's spiritual system, and latterly his healing system.

When we practise Reiki we are working with earth ki and heavenly ki, in a conscious or unconscious fashion; when we channel Reiki, we are channelling either the ki of earth or heaven, because that is what we are.

But Usui Sensei's system goes further than just acknowledging our true nature, our physical and spiritual nature, because Reiki allows us to fully experience our physical reality, and fully experience our spiritual essence. This is a powerful method for achieving balance.

We can return to that state of perfection we enjoyed at birth, before life corrupted us; we can be reborn.

Earth and heaven in the original Reiki system

How this was achieved is as follows: At second degree in the original system the student would be shown how to experience earth ki and heavenly ki, they would learn to 'become' the energies of earth and heaven. How this was achieved very much depended on the student's background, since Usui Sensei varied his teachings and methods according to the needs of his students.

If the student had a Buddhist background then they would have used meditations, and if they had a Shinto background then they would have chanted sacred sounds called 'kotodama'.

Later on in Usui's system, symbols were introduced for the Imperial Officers, but all these approaches had the same end in mind: to fully assimilate, to fully experience or become the energies of earth and heaven, the essence of what we are.

The meditations, the kotodama, and the symbols are all tools used to trigger, to invoke within us, to allow us to experience an energy or a state. Second degree is all about getting to grips with earth ki and heavenly ki, to fully assimilate those energies, to reconnect to what is within and realise our true nature.

Earth, heaven and the Reiki symbols

CKR and SHK represent earth ki and heavenly ki respectively, but they do not represent something new: these two energies are already within us. They do not represent something additional that we are connected to: they emphasise or flag up something that is already there.

Now, Usui Sensei's students worked long and hard to assimilate or integrate these energies. The might have spent 6-9 months just meditating on one energy, before moving on, so there were no short-cuts and it was a long process. They started with the energy of earth and moved on to work with the energy of heaven.

We can echo that original practice by working with the energies of CKR and SHK. It is not enough to be 'attuned' to a symbol – whatever that means – and it is not enough to use a symbol in practice when treating someone.

To fully get to grips with an energy we need to meditate on the symbol, using its energy individually, not combined with others, and we need to commit ourselves to doing this regularly if we are going to fully experience the benefits that are available through Usui Sensei's simple spiritual system.

Do I always have to use the symbols?

So many Reiki rules!

In most Reiki lineages the Reiki symbols are taught on the Second Degree course, though some are taught one symbol at First Degree I believe.

A lot of rules have built up about what you can and can't do with symbols, what you always must do, and of course these rules end up being contradictory.

The only rule that applies to Reiki is 'there are no rules' I believe, and what I'd like to do here is just run through a few 'symbol rules' that you can choose to ignore.

Draw the symbols over your palm every day or you'll "lose" them

Some poor Reiki people are frantically drawing the three symbols over their palms every morning because if they don't they'll "lose" the symbols and won't be able to use them any more.

I have to say that this is nonsense, and is something that most Reiki people will not be doing.

The symbols are graphical representations of different aspects of the energy, they are triggers that you can use to access and energy, to direct an energy, and you don't even need to be 'attuned' to a symbol for it to work for you (but that's another story).

Please don't draw the symbols over your palms every day for fear of losing them.

You always have to use the symbols when you treat

Why? Why would you always have to use the symbols when you treat someone?

You are attuned to Reiki, you have been working happily with the energy since your First Degree course, channelling it for your benefit and for the benefit of others, and suddenly someone does some mystical hand-waving over you and you can't use Reiki unless you keep drawing out symbols?

That makes no sense at all, particularly when you realise that there are a lot of Reiki practitioners and Masters who have moved away from, or beyond, the use of the symbols and just allow the energy to do what it needs to.

The symbols are useful tools, a way of focusing your attention on and experiencing different aspects of the energy, but they're not compulsory!

Try only using a symbol during a treatment when the symbol seems to 'want' to be used, when you feel it's right to use in a particular hand position, when it 'calls' to you.

Go with the flow and let the energy guide you, so you're gearing the treatment more towards the needs of the person you're working on.

See what happens.

Always draw every symbol over each hand position

Oh dear, this would be so ham-fisted, to have to frantically draw out three symbols in every hand position you use when treating someone.

If you were taught to do this, I would like to suggest that you experiment, try out different ways of working that don't involve this very busy, cluttered approach, and come to your own conclusions about what's necessary.

It's not a very Japanese approach, is it?

If you think about traditional Japanese arts they do pare things to the bone, leaving only the bare, elegant essentials.

Clutter-free Reiki is a much calmer, and potent.

Over to you

If you have been taught some of the rules and restrictions I mentioned above, please do experiment for yourself and come to your own conclusions about what's necessary and effective.

You don't need to slavishly follow all the instructions that you were given by your teacher; you can find your own comfortable approach with the energy.

Reiki Symbols, Attunements and Beyond

In the Western style of Reiki, the Reiki symbols are seen to be very important. They are seen as an integral part of the system; indeed for many people the symbols **are** Reiki, the symbols **are** the energy. It has been a basic tenet of Western Reiki that you have to be 'attuned' to the symbols for them to work for you and that you are connected to Reiki only when you have been 'attuned' to the symbols.

All Western style attunement systems – as far as I can see – involve being attuned to symbols at First Degree, Second Degree and Master levels. However, no one really knew if you needed to be attuned to the symbols for them to work for you, and no one really knew whether symbols needed to enter into the connection ritual used, because no one knew of a way to attune people without using symbols! The only connection rituals that we had were attunements, and all attunements used symbols!

But new information coming from Japan, and the experiences of some Reiki people experimenting in the West, suggest that the Reiki symbols might not be such a necessary part of 'attuning' people as was once thought, and suggest that there is no need for a person to be 'attuned' to a symbol for it to work for them, so long as they are already connected to Reiki.

Mikao Usui did not attune people

Now we now know that Mikao Usui did not teach symbols to the vast majority of his students, and those few students who were taught symbols (the Imperial Officers) were not 'attuned' to these symbols by Usui Sensei. In fact, Mikao Usui did not attune anybody to anything: he used to 'empower' his students, and the empowerments that he bestowed on his students, at all levels, did not utilise the Reiki symbols.

So where did attunements come from, and where did the idea of 'attuning' someone to symbols in order for the student to be 'connected' to Reiki, and to be able to use those symbols, come from?

Well it seems certain that the Imperial Officers had not trained with Usui Sensei for long enough before he died for them to have been taught by him how to empower students (Usui taught this quite far along on the Master student's journey). Usui did not attune people and he did not teach attunements.

It seems that the Imperial Officers developed for themselves a ritual – an 'attunement' - by way of trying to replicate the experiences that they had had when being empowered by Usui Sensei, and because they had been taught symbols, these symbols entered into the ritual that they developed.

A version of this ritual was passed from Dr Hayashi (one of the Imperial Officers) to Mrs Takata, who passed on a ritual to her Master students, and the ritual has now been endlessly distorted and embellished as it has been passed from teacher to teacher in the West.

Interestingly, Hiroshi Doi – a member of the Usui Reiki Ryoho Gakkai (Usui Memorial Society, set up after his death by some of the Imperial Officers) – has said that the 'attunement' methods used in the 'Gakkai do not involve the use of symbols: the 'Gakkai's students are connected to Reiki, but the Reiki symbols are not used in this process.

Mr Doi also said that Mikao Usui introduced the symbols for the benefit of students who could just not accept that they could 'do this thing', and by giving them something concrete to use, they learned to focus and control the energy more easily.

Hiroshi Doi also says that the current 'Gakkai students do not use the Reiki symbols, though they are shown them out of historical interest. Mikao Usui no doubt chose the symbols very carefully, to represent different aspects of the energy, but the energy and the connection to the energy came first.

Let's go back to the empowerments that Usui was using: the empowerments bestowed by Usui Sensei could be referred to as "Reiju", a Tendai Buddhist blessing made with the intention that the student should 'receive what they need', and a form of Reiju has been passed to us via Mikao Usui's surviving students.

Reiju is a way of 'connecting' you to Reiki, though all such rituals really do (whether attunements of empowerments) is to help you recognise something that is already there: they do not connect you to something external to you that you were not connected to before.

Reiju – at all levels – does not involve using symbols, at all. So Reiju is a way of 'connecting' someone to Reiki but without any symbols entering into the process. And thus we have a way of demonstrating, for the first time, that 'attuning' someone to a symbol is not a necessary step in 'connecting' them to Reiki.

This is quite a revelation for the world of Western-style Reiki.

Not only that, but now that we know how to connect people to Reiki without using symbols, and without 'attuning' people to symbols, we can at last find out whether one needs to be attuned to a symbol for it to work for us.

My experimentation

Many years ago I experimented...

I found, for example, that students attuned at First Degree level, using Western-style attunements, can produce noticeable effects in their hands when using the Reiki symbols; they can use the symbols, experience their energies and channel the energies that the symbols represent.

Western-style Reiki First Degree attunements use the Reiki symbols, of course, but you are not usually 'attuned' to them in the way that you are at Second Degree level, and First Degree students are not 'supposed' to be able to use the Reiki symbols, or carry out things like distant healing (though, of course, this is nonsense).

I also found that the symbols work just as well for First Degree students who are connected to Reiki using Reiju empowerments, (the symbol-free connection ritual). In fact, I have noticed that students attuned using Reiju seem to be more sensitive to the flow of Reiki than students attuned in the Western style.

Taking this one stage further, I have been using Reiju empowerments with students at Second Degree level, students who were 'connected' using Reiju at First Degree too, and found that students attuned in this way can use the Reiki symbols in just the same way, and just as effectively, as students attuned using the Western system... although these students have not been 'attuned' to the symbols.

You don't need to be "attuned" to a symbol

All this leads me to believe that once you have been connected to Reiki – and we now know that symbols do not need to enter into this process – then the Reiki symbols will work for you, and you do not need to be 'attuned' to them specifically (whatever that means).

Not only that, but I believe that **any** symbol will direct the energy in a particular way once you have been attuned to Reiki: Usui's chosen symbols which come from Shintoism and Tendai Buddhism, but also symbols from other cultures and traditions, and channelled symbols too.

I have personal experience of this, and so do my students.

Channelled symbols, for example, can be used effectively by people who have not been 'attuned' to them; they can be shown them, meditate on them and experience their characteristic energies. I have been in contact with a Moldovan Doctor (and Reiki Master) whose Reiki friends use Christian symbols to control and focus the Reiki energy.

I also know a Moslem Reiki Master who uses Moslem prayers to frame the energy in a particular way, and he can feel the energy altering its nature as the prayer is recited.

In Usui Sensei's original system, sacred sounds called 'kotodama' were taught as a way of experiencing, and directing, the energy. Students were not 'attuned' to a kotodama (however that might have been achieved): they simply used the sound and the sound moulded the energy.

The Reiki symbols are simply graphical representations of different aspects of the energy. You can simply look at them, remember them and use them and they will work for you, whether or not you have been through some sort of ritual that involved the teacher visualising them as they 'connected' you.

From personal experience, and the experience of many Reiki people, I can say that it is possible to produce the desired effect with the energy through intent only, whether that be distant healing or gearing the energy in the direction of mental/emotional balancing or physical healing.

So for me there is a distinction to be made between the energy of Reiki and any graphics (symbols) that might be used to control and focus the energy in a particular way. Reiki is the energy, you are 'connected' to the energy, but symbols do not need to enter into the connection process for it to work, nor do you need to have been 'attuned' to a symbol before it will work for you.

There are many ways of directing the energy: by using symbols from Japan or from other cultures or sources, by using sound, and through simple intent.

Simplicity and Sandwiches

In the West, there seems to be this insidious tendency to make things unnecessarily complicated, almost on the basis that if it's more complicated, it is better.

We have to take things and make them bigger and better; we have to add stuff.

In Japan, of course, they seem to go in the opposite direction, paring things down to the bone, getting rid of any unnecessary frills and flounces, leaving us with the pure essence of a thing, simple and elegant. Think of Japanese garden design, flower arranging, the tea ceremony, and you will see what I mean.

This contrast can be seen in the practices of Western Reiki and original Japanese Reiki.

Western attunements

Western attunements, for example, tend to be quite complicated affairs. There are lots of different Western ways of connecting you to Reiki, some of them quite contradictory in terms of the way that they are supposed to work, but they do all work.

Some have lots of puffing and blowing; some are more restrained. Some have lots of tapping and patting, others don't, some attune your hands, and some attune your fingertips. Some have different rituals at Reiki1, Reiki2 and Master levels, while others have exactly the same rituals but you repeat the process a different number of times at the different levels.

They all involve your head: they are busy, you are drawing symbols, saying names, putting things in different places, saying various affirmations in your head and imagining things.

Japansese empowerments

The Japanese approach is rather different. The way that Mikao Usui empowered people was simplicity itself, and his surviving students are passing on a simple, elegant connection ritual called 'Reiju", which is a way of conveying what Usui Sensei bestowed on his students.

Reiju is the same in its form at all levels and is a lovely energy dance, rather like following the flowing form of Tai Chi or Qigong. Reiju is not a 'head' activity, because you simply merge yourself with the energy and follow the form. It is a real pleasure to carry out, as anyone who has learned it will attest. Reiju is pure simplicity.

Hand positions for Reiki treatments

In some Western lineages there are rigid sets of hand positions that you have to follow, in all treatments. Some people are taught that not only must they always use these 'correct' hand positions, but they must also spend a set amount of time in each hand position.

They move their hands like robots from one position to another on hearing a 'bell' on one of a number of special CDs used as a guide.

Yet Usui's method took a simpler approach: rather than following a standard set of hand positions, you were expected to work at developing your intuition so that your hands were moved by the energy to the right places to treat.

The hand positions you used would change from one person to another, and from one treatment to another within the same person, based on their individual energy needs; a simple and elegant approach, free from dogma and rigidity.

The Reiki symbols

But it is in the use of the Reiki symbols, the Reiki energies, where there is perhaps the greatest gulf between Usui's original method and the techniques used in the West. In the West, Second Degree Reiki involves being 'attuned' to three symbols, two that can be used when giving treatments and a third used in the 'sending' of Reiki long-distance.

These were not 'new' symbols that were introduced to the world by Usui after a moment of enlightenment, as the Mrs Takata-inspired history of Reiki tells us, but existing symbols that he appropriated into his system quite late in Reiki's history.

Depending on what lineage we have, we are taught different ways of using these symbols. In one lineage you may be taught to use all three symbols in each and every hand position when you are treating someone. Another lineage will tell you that the second symbol is hardly ever to be used, or is only to be used in a narrow and predefined set of circumstances.

In most lineages the first symbol is seen as some sort of 'power' symbol that doesn't seem to do much on its own but makes other symbols stronger, and you are taught to put the symbols on top of each other, or mix them together.

Some people have developed quite complicated arrangements where you use one symbol, and then put another on top, and then another one, and then another one, and so on. This technique has been called the 'Reiki sandwich'. But are these approaches an unnecessary complication, and could there be a simpler approach that might be more effective in practice?

We Westerners seem to focus more on the Reiki symbols than in Japan. For example, according to Hiroshi Doi, the Usui Reiki Ryoho Gakkai ('Usui's Reiki Healing Association') does not use the Reiki symbols. Students are shown the symbols out of historical interest, but they are expected to work directly with the energies that the symbols represent.

We also know that most of the people that Mikao Usui taught were not given symbols, but used other approaches to connect to the energies that in the West we use the symbols to represent.

What is interesting too is the way that Usui had his students use these energies, because it challenges the Western way of using symbols. Rather than being some sort of 'power symbol', the first energy was seen as focusing on the physical body, it was seen as a physical healing energy.

This was the solid energy of earth.

The second energy was seen as producing harmony, it was celestial energy, working on the thoughts and emotions, the energy of our spiritual essence, a bit like the second symbol/energy is seen in the West.

So now we have energies that will deal with healing the body, and the mind / emotions / spirit, the whole spectrum.

Not only that, but these energies were used individually, on their own, not mixed endlessly with other energies and symbols in complicated arrangements and sequences.

You chose an energy using your intuition, and you focused on it. By focusing on one thing, rather than trying to do lots of things at the same time, you intensify the effect.

Isn't that simple?

A Simple Way with Symbols

In the West we like to make things complicated, and the way that most of us now use symbols is a world away from the simple approach that Usui used. So how can we work with symbols in a way that echoes more the way that Usui taught his students?

Well firstly, Usui taught symbols to a very small number of people, just in the last few years of his life. The vast majority of his students were taught in a very different way. Most of his students were given meditations to use so that they could, over a long period of time, become more and more familiar with the three energies taught at second-degree level, for example.

Once they were thoroughly familiar with the energies, once they had *become* the energies again and again, then they were given a shortcut – a trigger – to connect them to those energies. The triggers that they used were ancient Shinto mantras called kotodama or jumon, not symbols.

In the West we do it backwards by comparison: we are given a trigger (a symbol) to connect us to an energy that we are not familiar with, and with which we may never become familiar, depending on how we have been taught to use the symbols.

Usui had his students become the three energies again and again and again, and when they were ingrained, when they were innate, only then would you be given a way of connecting to the energies that were already within you and thoroughly familiar to you.

The energies were also viewed somewhat differently. The first energy was not seen as some sort of 'Power' energy, in the way that the first symbol is seen as the 'Power' symbol in the West. The first energy was simply earth energy, energy of the physical body, a physical healing energy.

The second energy was seen as heavenly energy and the third energy was said to produce 'oneness'. Usui's students learned to get to grips with these energies through meditation, so how can we learn to experience earth energy and celestial energy? Well, we can do this by using the symbols…

Try this simple energy exercise

St comfortably in a chair with your eyes closed and your hands resting in your lap palms uppermost. In your mind's eye, visualise the first symbol up in the air above you, and say its name silently to yourself three times.

Now imagine that cascades of energy are flooding down onto you from that symbol, cascading into your head, your torso, your hands; endless cascades of energy or light keep on flooding into your body, flowing over you and flooding through you. Do this for several minutes.

How does that feel? What impressions do you get of the energy? Where was your attention focused? What were your thoughts?

Now repeat this exercise using the second symbol, again visualising it up in the air above you, saying its name three times, and drawing down endless cascades of energy into your body.

How does this feel by comparison? What impressions do you get of the second energy? Where is your attention focused? What is going on in your head?

Try this exercise with a partner

If you have a Reiki friend to hand, you can do this exercise together: one person sits comfortably in a chair and the other stands behind. The person standing up is going to send energy from the first or second symbol in quite an intense way.

What they do is this: 'charge' your hands with the energy of the first symbol, say, by drawing the symbol over your palm, saying the name three times, and press your hands together to 'transfer the effect across' to he other hand.

Now in your mind's eye draw out the first symbol up in the air above you and say the name three times. Move your hands so that they are hovering alongside the recipient's temples, and imagine that you are drawing down cascades of energy from the symbol above you, which flood into your crown, through your arms and out of your hands into the recipient.

Keep on visualising.

How does the energy feel as it comes through your hands? What impressions do you get in your body? How does it feel for the recipient? What adjectives can they use to describe the essence of the energy that they have received?

Now repeat this exercise using the second symbol. How does this differ from the first energy?

Having carried out this exercise countless times and with many, many students, I can generalise about the sort of impression that most people tend to get from the two symbols, the two energies. Maybe you will notice some, though not all, of these experiences.

The first energy seems thick, dark, heavy, dense, solid, maybe oppressive or claustrophobic sometimes, hot, fierce, coarse, penetrating, with pressure and slow pulsation, your focus is on your physical body. The second energy seems soft, light, gentle, ethereal, like soft fluffy clouds or marshmallows, cool, blue, expansive, exhilarating, and uplifting.

What you have experienced is the essence of earth energy and the essence of heavenly energy, and these are two energies that you have available to you when treating others.

These energies are the essence of Usui's system at second-degree level. The first energy focuses on the physical body, and the second focuses on thoughts and emotions and our spiritual nature. They are so different, so distinctive.

Try using them on their own, just one energy, just one focus, without mixing symbols together. Keep things simple and uncluttered by focusing like a laser beam on one thing at a time, and see what happens. And with time, and with familiarity with the two energies, try producing those energies directly, using intent, and see what happens.

Were you taught the correct "Power" symbol: variations on CKR

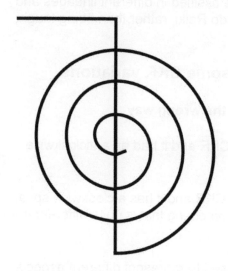

Reiki started simply

Reiki is very simple, you know.

You start working with energy at First Degree and at Second Degree you're introduced to three symbols that you can use.

These symbols were taught to the Imperial Officers and a few others by Usui Sensei, and Dr Hayashi passed them on to Mrs Takata, who taught them in the West.

One of those symbols was CKR, perfect and complete on itself – see above.

So we started messing about with it, which is fine – experimentation is a good thing – but some of the experiments have become ossified in different lineages and passed on as 'the' way to do Reiki, rather than being taught as interesting variations.

Let's have a look at some CKR variations

CKR with a spiral going the wrong way

There was only ever one CKR and it had an anticlockwise spiral.

If you've been taught one CKR and it has a clockwise spiral then you've been taught something that is quite different from what Usui intended.

Different shapes can be used to represent different aspects of the energy, and they will all frame the energy in a particular way.

If you want to frame the energy in the way that Usui intended then you do need to use the symbol that he taught.

Use two mirror-image CKRs, not one

There was only ever one CKR and it had an anticlockwise spiral, so if you want to use an additional symbol that is a mirror image of the original then that's your choice, but please realise that this is not what Usui was teaching and most Reiki people don't do this.

Certainly don't feel that you 'have' to use these two symbols for Reiki to work properly because that simply isn't the case.

Use CKR to put energy in and reverse CKR to take energy out

CKR is an image that you can use to represent or elicit earth ki, one of the two basic energies or aspects of our existence: earth ki and heavenly ki.

The person who you are working on will draw that energy to where they need it to go, and in the right amounts for them on that occasion. If you're stepping in to decide for yourself that they need more energy or less energy, you aren't really allowing the energy to do what it needs to do, unless you are doing this intuitively, in which case you're working in partnership with the energy, and it is guiding you.

Usui Sensei didn't teach two CKRs, one of them to take out energy; there was a reason for that: Reiki will do what people need to have done, and if energy needs to be released then plain Reiki will help a person with that without you having to use a specific symbol to achieve it.

If you are currently using a reverse-CKR to 'take out energy', you might try dispensing with that for a while and see what happens.

So if you want to use the variations on CKR then that's your choice, but please know that while this is **a** way that you can work with Reiki, it is not **the only** way, other Reiki people work in a different way from you, and these variations were not part of the system that Usui taught.

Over to you

If you were taught some of these non-standard versions of CKR as "the" way that you should practise Reiki, may I suggest that you experiment:

- Use the CKR that you can see on this page, meditate on its energy to get to grips with how it feels, how it affects you
- Draw it over your palm to experience its energy
- Use it in practice when you treat someone, flooding yourself and your client with its energy

How is what you're doing different in quality or nature from what you were doing before?

Some heresy about Reiki symbols

You don't need to be attuned to a symbol

In my article, "Reiki Symbols, Attunements & Beyond", I explain that although it has been a belief of traditional Western Reiki that the Reiki symbols will not work for you until you have been specifically 'attuned' to them, this belief is not correct.

I suggest that you zip across and read that article now because if you do then this article here will make more sense to you!

I'll wait...

.

.

.

Done?

OK, so we have a situation in the modern Reiki world where people can now be initiated into Reiki without any symbols entering into the process and, when that happens, the Reiki symbols – CKR, SHK – still work fine, eliciting the energies of earth ki and heavenly ki, as they are supposed to.

The 'attunement' thing isn't a necessary step.

The energy can be focused and modified in many different ways: you can use chants, you can use intent and you can use *any* symbol that you like, whether that's a symbol from one of the many Reiki variations, or an entirely new, channelled, or random symbol. They will all focus or frame the energy in a particular way.

Let's experiment with some symbols

So if you feel drawn to, say, Karuna Reiki, which is heavily symbol-based, and you have access to the symbols used in that system, then explore its symbols. Meditate on them, draw their energies into your body, flood yourself with their quality or essence, and come to your own conclusion about what they are all about.

Here's a simple experiment that you an carry out to prove to yourself that a symbol that you haven't been attuned to will frame the energy in a distinctive way.

Meditation on "O"

I would like you to meditate on a simple circle. Rest your hands in your lap, palms up, close your eyes and take a couple of long, deep breaths to release any stress and tension.

Then imagine a perfect circle, black & white, up in the air above you. Imagine that energy or light is cascading down to you from that symbol above you, flooding over you, flowing through you, and just bathe in that energy, merging with it.

Here's an example for you:

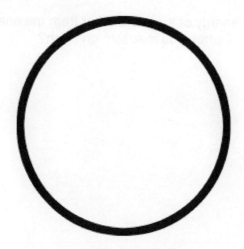

Alternatively, meditate in time with your breath so that on the inbreath you draw energy down from that circle into your tanden, allow the energy to flow and spread through your body, and on the outbreath just flood that energy out of you.

And notice how that energy feels:

- Where do you feel it most?
- What quality does it have?
- What impression do you have of its nature?
- What does it do to/for you?
- What is its essence?

Over to you

Carry out the meditation a few times and post a message below to let me know what the energy of the circle felt like.

What did it do for you?

How did the energy of the circle differ from the energies of CKR and SHK when you meditate on them?

Let's explore some non-Reiki symbols

Where we are now

In my article "Some heresy about Reiki symbols" I explained that you do not need to be 'attuned' to a symbol for that symbol to work for you when you're channelling the energy, and that any symbol – wherever it came from – will frame and focus the Reiki energy in a distinctive way.

I set you the exercise of meditating on a simple circle, putting the symbol up in the air above you and drawing Reiki down from that symbol, to flood over you and through you.

You were meditating on and experiencing "O" flavour Reiki, or circle-flavour Reiki.

Let's explore some more simple symbols

This week I would like you to experiment with two more symbols, a **triangle** and a **square**. Meditate on each one for 5 minutes or so.

This is what to do: rest your hands in your lap with palms up, close your eyes and take a couple of deep breaths to release any tension.

Then imagine a perfect triangle – an equilateral – black & white, up in the air above you. Imagine that energy or light is flooding to you from the symbol above you, cascading over you, flowing through you, and bathe in that energy; feel yourself merging with it.

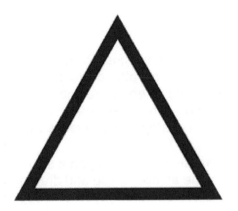

Alternatively, meditate in time with your breath so that on the inbreath you draw energy down from that circle into your tanden, allow the energy to flow and spread through your body, and on the outbreath just flood that energy out of you.

And notice how that energy feels:

- Where do you feel it most?
- What quality does it have?
- What impression do you have of its nature?
- What does it do to/for you?
- What is its essence?

Now repeat the exercise using the square.

Go back to the "O" and remind yourself how that felt.

Over to you

Carry out the meditation a few times and post a message below to let me know what the energy of the triangle and square felt like.

What did they do for you?

How did the energy of the triangle and the square differ from the energies of "O" and how were they different from CKR and SHK when you meditate on them? You're quite sensitive to the energy, aren't you?

Create your own bespoke Reiki symbols

Create symbols tailor made for you

I have written several articles dealing with Reiki symbols and how you don't need to be attuned to a symbol for it to 'work' for you , and that *any* symbol will frame the energy when you focus your attention on it or meditate on it.

It might be useful if you quickly re-visit these articles because they will help with this article:

- Reiki symbols, attunements and beyond
- Some heresy about Reiki symbols
- Let's explore some non-Reiki symbols

So wouldn't it be great if it was possible for you to create a symbol that framed the energy in just the 'perfect' way for you, now, this day?

Wouldn't it be something if you could use a symbol that gives you just what you need in this moment, in a powerful and profound way, framing the energy in *just* the way that you need, focused like a laser-beam?

Well this is possible and in this article I am going to explain how to do this.

Using the "if" question to create a bespoke Reiki symbol

To create a symbol that will frame the energy in a way that perfectly matches your needs, you can use these three questions, which you ask yourself:

1. **If** the energy that I need in this moment had a **shape**, what shape would it be?
2. **If** it had a colour, what **colour** would it be?
3. **If** that energy was to be held in a particular part of my **body**, where would it be held?

Allow the answers to come to you; go with the first thing that comes into your mind.

So now you have, say, a green star that needs to reside in your abdomen (I have chosen this at random).

Now use the symbol that you have been given

Rest your hands in your lap, palms up, close your eyes and take a couple of long, deep breaths to release any stress and tension.

Imagine that shape in that colour, up in the air above you, representing the source of the energy (this is just like the symbol meditations that we teach on the Reiki Evolution Second Degree course). Imagine energy of that colour flooding down to you from the symbol above you, focusing/drawing the energy into that part of your body (in this example, the abdomen).

Feel the energy in that location and allow that colour to flood through your whole body.

Experience that energy for a few minutes.

You could, of you like, imagine that the coloured symbol is actually passing into that location in your body, as that coloured energy continues to flow down to you from that symbol above you.

No good at visualising? No problem

If you're not so good at visualizing at the moment, focus not so much on the shape of the symbol, but the feel of it, the texture or density: feel the shape rather than seeing it; if you can't see the colour very well, simply intend or 'know' that the shape and the energy has that particular hue.

In doing so, you and embodying the essence of that energy.

As a variation, you might draw the energy to your Tanden as you inhale, breathing the energy to its chosen location on the out-breath; experiment and find out what works best for you.

Why do I ask "If..."?

You are asking your subconscious mind a question about the best way to represent the energy that you need and this works best if you don't put too much 'pressure' on your mind to come up with the goods.

If you said "what shape is the energy I need" your unconscious might have some performance anxiety and start fretting about things, essentially saying "what do you mean

what 'shape'... I don't know, that's difficult, how am I
supposed to know that, what do you mean "shape"?... don't
hassle me".

By framing the question in terms of "if..." you are taking the
pressure off.

It's as if you're saying to yourself "I'm not saying that this
energy does have a shape... but **if it did**, what would that
shape be? No pressure."

Over to you

What I would like you to do is to go through those three
questions and when you have the answer, meditate on the
energy that comes from that symbol/shape for about 10
minutes.

Create a bespoke Reiki symbol for your client

Create symbols tailor made for your clients

In my last Reiki article, "Create your own bespoke Reiki symbols", I described a simple system that you can follow in order to create a Reiki symbol that provides you with an energy perfectly suited to just what you need in this moment.

And we know that using a symbol has the effect of focusing the Reiki energy like a laser beam, narrowing its focus and boosting its power.

So this would be a useful thing to be able to do for clients too, wouldn't it, to give them a treatment that uses an energy ideally suited to just what they need in this moment?

Here is how to do that.

Asking some questions of your unconscious mind

Settle yourself at the head of the treatment table, say, and rest your hands on your client's shoulders. I think it's nice to start a treatment like this, getting the energy flowing, helping them to bliss out.

Imagine that you are merging with the energy and the recipient. Start to bliss out yourself!

With your attention focused on the recipient, say to yourself ask yourself:

1. **If** the energy that this person needs in this moment had a **shape**, what shape would it be?
2. **If** it had a colour, what **colour** would it be?
3. **If** that energy was to be held in a particular part of **their body**, where would it be held?

Allow the answers to come to you; go with the first thing that comes into your mind.

So now you have, say, an attractive blue 3D spiral that needs to reside in their solar plexus (I have chosen this at random).

Flood your client with this energy

So now you know that the energy your client needs in this moment is best represented for you as a 3D blue spiral that wants to focus itself in their solar plexus.

Now you can start to use this energy and you can do that in two ways (or both).

With your hands still resting on their shoulders...

Imagine that shape in that colour, up in the air above you, representing the source of the energy. Imagine energy of that colour flooding down to you from the symbol above you, flowing through your shoulders, arms and hands, flowing into the client.

Have in mind that the energy is flowing into their solar plexus. Focus your attention there and imagine that the energy is dwelling there.

You could, of you like, imagine that the coloured symbol is actually passing into that location in their body, as that coloured energy continues to flow down to you from that symbol above you.

Or later on during the treatment…

When you get to the torso, rest your hands on or near their solar plexus, or hover your hands over that area, and follow the instructions above: draw down that colour energy from that symbol above you, which flows through your arms and hands, while focusing your attention on and treating the solar plexus.

No good at visualising? No problem

If you're not so good at visualizing at the moment, focus not so much on the shape of the symbol, but the feel of it, the texture or density: feel the shape rather than seeing it; if you can't see the colour very well, simply intend or 'know' that the shape and the energy has that particular hue.

In doing so, you and embodying the essence of that energy.

As a variation, you might draw the energy to your Tanden as you inhale, breathing the energy out of your hands into its chosen location on the out-breath; experiment and find out what works best for you.

Over to you

What I would like you to do is to go through those three
questions when you work on a client or friend or family
member, and when you have the answer, channel the energy
that comes from that symbol/shape for about 10 minutes into
the area of the body where the energy wants to go.

The simplest distant healing method ever!

Lets' explore Reiki distant healing

What I would like to do in a series of articles is to suggest some different DH approaches. Some may be familiar to you; some may be new.

If you discover a new approach then try it for yourself and see how it feels, and come to your own conclusion about what seems the best way for you, the most comfortable 'fit'.

Distant healing is a very important part of Reiki practice, of course, and is something that is not unique to Reiki. Distant healing (DH for short) is carried out in different Reiki lineages in different ways and there is no one 'right' way to perform this process.

The important thing when carrying out DH is your underlying intent, and the details of the ritual that you use are unimportant.

Simplest distant healing method ever!

What I would like to share with you today is probably just about the simplest version of DH that you can find (I may be wrong here!). It doesn't involve symbols, it doesn't involve complex imagery or long affirmations.

It cuts things down to their bare bones, the essence of DH.

How to do distance healing with Reiki

The bare bones of distant healing are to know where you are sending the energy – to set a definite intent – and to allow the energy to flow, so you could try this:

1. Close your eyes and take a few long deep breaths
2. Focus your attention on your Tanden point
3. Say to yourself that "this is to be a distant healing for the highest good of ....[the person's name]"
4. Focus your attention on the recipient in your mind's eye/imagination
5. Feel yourself merging with the recipient, becoming one with them
6. Allow the energy to flow from you to them for as long as feels appropriate
7. When you are ready to bring things to a close, feel your attention withdrawing from the recipient by way of 'disconnecting' from them, take a few long deep breaths again, and bring yourself back

In this example we dedicated the distant healing to the recipient's highest good, which means that we were neutral in the process, not directing the energy to achieve a particular result.

We approach distant healing in the same way that we approach treating another person: we have no expectations, we stand aside and we allow the energy to do whatever is appropriate for that person.

The energy is drawn through us according to the recipient's need without any interference from us; we have no thought or desire about the outcome

Distant healing with imagined hand positions

A very simple distant healing method

What I would like to share with you today is another simple version of DH.

It doesn't involve symbols, it doesn't involve complex imagery or long affirmations, though it does involve some imagining. This method cuts the process down to its essential parts.

Distance healing with imagined hand positions

The bare bones of distant healing are to know where you are sending the energy – to set a definite intent – and to allow the energy to flow, and as you do that, it can be helpful to imagine something to help maintain your focus, or to focus your intent.

So you could try this:

1. Close your eyes and take a few long deep breaths
2. Focus your attention on your Tanden point
3. Say to yourself that "this is to be a distant healing for the highest good of ….[the person's name]"
4. Imagine that the recipient is sitting on the floor in front of you
5. Feel yourself merging with the recipient, becoming one with them
6. In your mind's eye, imagine or have in mind that the energy is flowing into the person's shoulders

7. Move on to imagine that you are going through a series of hand positions on the person's head; go with whatever feels right or appropriate
8. Finish with the shoulders again.
9. When you are ready to bring things to a close, feel your attention withdrawing from the recipient by way of 'disconnecting' from them, take a few long deep breaths again, and bring yourself back

In this example we dedicated the distant healing to the recipient's highest good, which means that we were neutral in the process, not directing the energy to achieve a particular result.

We approach distant healing in the same way that we approach treating another person: we have no expectations, we stand aside and we allow the energy to do whatever is appropriate for that person.

The energy is drawn through us according to the recipient's need without any interference from us; we have no thought or desire about the outcome

Over to you

If this approach is new to you, why not try it and see how you get on.

Distant healing with a little bit of ritual attached

Distant healing is a very important part of Reiki practice, of course, and is something that is not unique to Reiki. Distant healing (DH for short) is carried out in different Reiki lineages in different ways and there is no one 'right' way to perform this process.

Distance healing made more of an "event"

The important thing when carrying out DH is your underlying intent, and the details of the ritual that you use are unimportant. What I would like to share with you today is a more complex version of DH.

Some people like more of an 'event' when they send distant healing, with the details of the ritual helping people to maintain their focus. The details aren't really so important, but if you like your rituals more 'High Church' than 'Low Church' then perhaps you'll like this version.

Remember that the bare bones of distant healing are to know where you are sending the energy – to set a definite intent – and to allow the energy to flow, and anything beyond that is personal preference.

Cup your hands together

Below is a method based on one used by my first Reiki teacher, Diane Whittle.

Basically you visualise the recipient and shrink them down so that they fit between your hands. Visualise the distant healing symbol over your hand to make a connection and let the energy flow; you can add CKR or SHK if you wish, as feels necessary.

I like to clear a space on my desk, light a candle and maybe some incense and just sit quietly for a while watching the candle flame and the plume of smoke from the incense stick. It helps me to relax and quieten my mind. It sets the scene for the ritual to follow.

This is what I do next:

1. Settle yourself down and blank your mind for a few moments.
2. Say to yourself that this is to be a distant healing for the highest healing good of [say recipient's name].
3. Visualise the person (if you know them) and imagine them as they might be in their usual surroundings, home etc. in order to make a connection with them.
4. Imagine the person being shrunk down so that they fit in the palm of your non-dominant hand.
5. Draw HonShaZeShoNen over the palm of your non-dominant hand, visualising the symbol in violet and saying its name three times.
6. Close your other hand over the top so that the person is 'cupped' between your hands.
7. Say to yourself' distant healing… connect' and imagine a tube of energy flowing from your cupped hands to the person you are treating, surrounding and engulfing their entire body with vibrant healing energy.
8. Visualise ChoKuRei or SeiHeKi as required, saying the symbol name three times, and imagine energy derived from that symbol flowing to the person.

9. Alternatively, just let the energy flow as it wants.
10. Perhaps imagine yourself carrying out a brief treatment on the person
11. Perhaps be creative: flood their body with brilliant white light, flushing away any negativity or disease; imagine some psychic surgery, reaching in and removing diseased parts.
12. You do not have to actively visualise; you can just let the Reiki flow.
13. Continue this for about 10-15 minutes
14. Finish by saying to yourself 'I seal this treatment with light and love and universal wisdom'. Intend that the healing effect is sealed in and that the benefits will be long-lasting.
15. Say to yourself 'distant healing... disconnect', visualising the energy tube disconnecting and disappearing.
16. Ritually disconnect as you would normally, rubbing or shaking your hands, blowing through them etc.

In this example we dedicated the distant healing to the recipient's highest good, which means that we were neutral in the process, not directing the energy to achieve a particular result.

We approach distant healing in the same way that we approach treating another person: we have no expectations, we stand aside and we allow the energy to do whatever is appropriate for that person.

The energy is drawn through us according to the recipient's need without any interference from us; we have no thought or desire about the outcome

Over to you

If this method is new to you, why not try it and see how you get on?

Distant healing using some sort of a prop

Distant healing is a very important part of Reiki practice, of course, and is something that is not unique to Reiki. Distant healing (DH for short) is carried out in different Reiki lineages in different ways and there is no one 'right' way to perform this process.

As you know, the important thing when carrying out DH is your underlying intent, and the details of the ritual that you use are unimportant.

What I would like to share with you today are some methods that use 'props' to represent the recipient.

Bears, pillows and legs

As a prop, you can use a teddy bear or other cuddly toy, and by sending Reiki into the teddy bear's head, or chest, or arm etc you are directing the energy to that part of the recipient, at a distance.

Some choose to use a pillow to represent the person, with one end of the pillow representing the recipient's head and the other end representing their feet.

Some people are taught to use their upper leg or legs to represent the person to whom distant healing is being sent, with your knee representing their head, and the part of your leg next to your hip representing their feet.

Some people use both legs, with one leg representing the front of the recipient, and the other leg representing the back of the recipient's body.

Props can help you focus

These props are there to help you to focus your attention, to focus your intent, and are not a necessary part of the process: distant healing can be carried out simply 'in your head', in a meditative state, but for those who like to have something tangible to work on, they can work very well, with the practitioner resting or hovering their hands over the different parts of the prop's 'body' and imagining that energy is flowing into that area, directing the energy into that part of the recipient's body at a distance.

Over to you

If these approaches are new to you, why not try them out and see how you get on

Do I need permission to send distant healing?

Is it unethical to send distant healing?

Some people are of the opinion that it is totally unethical to send distant Reiki to a person if they have not given their permission first.

They see it as a gross intrusion, interference, a violation of that person's personal space, a violation of their energy field. I do not agree with this point of view and I see no problem in sending Reiki to whoever you want.

Here are my reasons…

Reiki is a beautiful healing energy that will not cause anyone any harm, and any Reiki sent is dedicated to the 'highest good' of the recipient, so that it is line with their karma or destiny.

This means that you are not manipulating them or imposing your preferred result on the situation: if the person really does not want to be healed, or it is not appropriate for them to benefit, then the Reiki will not work.

Permission to pray?

You do not obtain someone's permission if you are going to pray for them, and I see sending distant healing rather like a concentrated form of prayer, where you are asking for Divine intervention in someone's life, in whatever way is appropriate for them.

Nobody rings up their friends to obtain their permission to pray for them. When there is a natural disaster somewhere in the world and people are praying for victims, they don't withold the prayer until they have obtained the written permission of all the faceless intended recipients.

If someone was lying in the road, unconscious after a road accident, would you refrain from sending Reiki to them just because they couldn't sit up and give you consent in writing? No, of course not: you'd send Reiki to their highest good and hope that it made a positive difference to them.

Scare stories about people being made to wake up when under an anaesthetic when receiving distant Reiki are just that – scare stories – like so many of the restrictions placed on people's Reiki practices because of myth and unfounded rumour. And if you are really worried that this might happen, then simply intend that the energy be received by the person at whatever moment is appropriate for them in the next 24 hours.

We are neutral in the process

We should remind ourselves that when we send distant Reiki we are neutral in the process, we have no expectations and we do not push for a particular outcome. We stand aside and what the energy does, if anything, is out of our hands. We offer the energy to the recipient, we do not force it on them, we do not make the energy do anything for the recipient; it is just there for them to use as they wish, or not. So permission is irrelevant.

Sending Reiki distant healing to the past

Getting creative with Reiki distant healing

I suppose that most people who send practise healing will send the energy to a friend or a family member, but the energy can be used more creatively too and, since Reiki doesn't seem greatly constrained by either time or space, some people will send Reiki to 'heal their past'.

They would do that by imagining a past situation or event which has had some ongoing effect on them in terms of what they believe about themselves, some event that has held them back in some way, preventing them from being the person they could be, and imagine that the energy is cradling or flooding that event, doing whatever needs to be done to bring healing and resolution.

Whether the energy actually flies back in time to flood that event with Reiki is a moot point I think, but since all we have to experience is the present in any case – we live in the now – what this practice does is to heal the ongoing effects that the earlier event has had on the way that we feel about ourselves and other people, for example; it calms the 'ripples' that the event has produced over the years, to remove the chains that are holding us back in some way.

Healing the 'inner child'

Some people might send distant healing to themselves in the past, imagining themselves as a child, by way of healing the 'inner child', not imagining a particular event or situation, but a representation or composite of them in childhood.

And, interestingly, this seems almost to be a Reiki version of 'Time Line' work, which is a practice in NLP: clients are taken back to find early events that have had a deleterious effect on their self-esteem, for example, and insights are passed on to the younger them that have knock-on effects in terms of how that earlier situation has affected them.

Over to you

If this idea is new to you, why not experiment and see what's possible?

Sending Reiki distant healing to the future

Using distant healing creatively

I suppose that most people who send practise healing will send the energy to a friend or a family member, but the energy can be used more creatively too and, since Reiki doesn't seem greatly constrained by either time or space, some people will send Reiki to their future.

So how might this be done?

Well, imagine that you have a public speaking engagement or a job interview, or a musical performance or an exam, any event where you could do with a bit of Reiki contentment sparkling over you. What you do is to imagine yourself in that future event, in whatever way feels comfortable, and imagine that Reiki is flooding into that event or situation, flooding into the room maybe, surrounding and engulfing you and any other people who might be there.

The Reiki that you are sending gives you just what you need on that occasion, supporting, nourishing and healing in the way that you need it, working its magic on the relationship between the people that are going to be there perhaps.

Reiki your day

Some people send Reiki 'to their day' by imagining their day ahead (in a brief, truncated or speeded up fashion) and flooding their day with Reiki, imagining everything going well, smoothly, calmly.

I have heard of someone who sends Reiki to 'their bed' each day, with the intention that the Reiki hangs around, ready to deposit itself on that person when they get into bed.

You can be endlessly creative with this!

Over to you

If this idea is new to you, why not experiment and see what's possible?

Ditch the dogma in Reiki distant healing

Find your own distant healing method

Distant healing is carried out in a huge number of ways in different lineages. There is endless variety.

Some methods are more complex than others, and some approaches are more dogmatic than others.

Some students are taught that if they do not carry out distant healing in a particular way then it will not work for them. This is unhelpful and Reiki is certainly not constrained by the details of man-made rituals.

What do we need for distant healing to succeed?

What does distant healing boil down to?

What are the essential steps?

Well, there are no hard and fast rules associated with distant healing, other than:

1. Knowing where the energy is going (setting a definite intent)
2. Using HSZSN in some way*
3. Allowing the energy to flow

*Even using HSZSN is actually optional, as you will have seen if you read my earlier "How to send Distant Healing" articles.

This lack of certainty can be rather disconcerting for some people, and liberating for others, so you can choose your method according to your taste. If you prefer simplicity, boil your approach down to barest essentials, or if you like a 'big event' then make your ritual more detailed, more 'High Church'.

So long as you know where you want the energy to go, and use HSZSN in some way if you want to, then the energy will get there.

You will find your own preferred technique

Remember that no one way is better than any other.

Some people feel more comfortable with a more detailed ritual, others are content to set a definite intent, use HSZSN to make the connection in some way, maybe, and they then blank their minds to allow the energy to flow, and visualise no longer.

Do what feels right for you.

Over to you

Is the way that you now practise Reiki distant healing different from how you were first taught?

How does what you do now differ? What method do you find most comfortable for you?

Distant healing, oneness and Mikao Usui's original system

Distant healing in Usui's time

Distant healing is an essential part of Reiki in the West. People on Second Degree courses are taught the 'distant healing' symbol and they learn how to 'send' Reiki to other people, in a way that transcends time and space.

But how was this done in Mikao Usui's time?

Well, it seems that distant healing was not practised by Usui Sensei's students, not in the way that we understand it, though they would have realised that such a thing was possible. And although we in the West are taught a 'distant healing symbol', these Reiki symbols were only introduced towards the end of Usui's life, for the benefit of the Imperial Officers who trained with him, and thus most of the people Usui trained were not give symbols to use.

Most of his students used either Buddhist-style meditations or chanted Shinto mantras called 'kotodama' to get to grips with certain energies and states, and the work that they were doing was all about their own spiritual development and self-healing; treating others was not focused on or emphasised in the original system for example, and neither was distant healing.

So if the original students weren't given HSZSN (the 'distant healing symbol') to use, and if they didn't practise distant healing, what did they do that ties in with the idea of distant healing?

Reiki and Oneness

It's all about Oneness, and this is a Buddhist idea: the concept that what we experience as reality is actually illusion, the idea that we are individuals, separate and distinct from other people is illusion, and that the true reality is that of oneness.

In Usui Sensei's original system, some Second Degree practitioners who had worked for up to 18 months with the energies of earth ki and heavenly ki were given the opportunity to meditate on and chant kotodama that elicited a state of oneness, one of the goals of the original system.

For me, practising distant healing is a good way to experience a state of oneness because in distant healing you are becoming one with the recipient, you merge with them and the energy and you lose that distinction between the sender and receiver, subject and object.

It's interesting that when we 'send' distant healing we are not sending and the receiver isn't receiving: the idea is that there is no us and there is no them, and that's why it's possible.

A lovely conundrum!

Over to you

When you practise distant healing, what do you notice about the state that you experience?

Do you find that you're in a space where you seem to transcend time and space?

What is your experience of oneness?

HSZSN but not as you've seen it before!

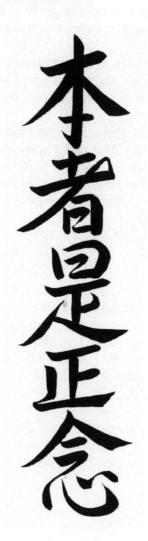

HSZSN is the acronym used to refer to the 'distant healing symbol', familiar in its various guises to anyone who has attended a Second Degree Reiki course.

It's the trickiest of the symbols to get to grips with and usually has 20+ strokes or hand movements to draw it out.

HSZSN actually consists of five separate Japanese kanji which have all been overlapped and merged to produce one 'composite' kanji, which we see on courses.

In this article I have posted an image of what these five separate kanji look like. The calligraphy was kindly brushed for me by the fantastically talented Japanese Calligraphy Shihan Eri Takase, who does all our Japanese writing for us, on our Reiki certificate templates, Reiki precepts prints, Reiki audio CDs and Reiki manuals.

Chinese whispers

When people attended Reiki courses in the past, many students and Masters weren't provided with hard copies of the Reiki symbols and so had to reproduce them from memory. That perhaps wasn't so bad for the simpler symbols like CKR and SHK, but for HSZSN this led to a process of "Chinese whispers", where the drawings altered slightly each time they were taught.

So now, quite understandably, there are various versions of the symbols in existence, some closer to and some really quite different from the original Japanese source.

Eri's calligraphy takes us back to the originals, though. It's great to see the original individual characters that the symbol was based on.

Merging the separate symbols

If you look at the image, you can see that the bottom part of the first kanji looks rather like the top part of the second kanji, so you could move the upper kanji downwards so that the 'cross' overlaps, producing one composite figure.

Similarly the bottom section of the second kanji looks rather like the top section of the third kanji, so they could be merged and overlapped. And so on down the line.

And that's how the composite HSZSN was formed!

Over to you

Have a look at the distant healing symbol that you were given.

See if you can work out what has changed, and what has stayed the same, compared to the original characters.

Working with Intuition

Intuition is available to everyone

When I first started practising Reiki, I didn't believe that I was intuitive. In fact, I thought that I might only be able to become intuitive after years of dedicated practice, if then. I thought that maybe intuition was only for the gifted few, or if it did arrive for me then it would flash into my head, gone in an instant, and I would not know how to get it back again.

I now realise that intuition is available for everyone, right from the word go, and that by doing just a few simple things we can all amaze ourselves with what we can become aware of.

Partly I have come to this conclusion through trial and error, and partly through practising an intuitive technique called 'Reiji ho' that is used in Japanese-style Reiki, a technique that allows your hands to be moved 'by invisible magnets' to the right places to treat. I have a long way to go with intuition: it is a lifelong journey, but I thought some people might find my experiences and experimentation interesting to read about…

Using a pendulum

For a while I used to use a pendulum when I treated people. I had agreed with the pendulum what it would do if a chakra was closed, spinning too fast, or 'normal', and I would dangle the pendulum over each chakra in turn and ask 'show me the state of the crown chakra', and so on along the length of the body.

Some people ask if each chakra in turn is balanced, others dangle the pendulum and watch its direction of rotation and size of circle traced out, showing how the chakra spins and how open it is. I found after a while that I did not need to hold the pendulum over the chakra; I could just hold the pendulum at my side and ask it as the client lay in front of me.

Then I discovered that I did not need to have the client in front of me either, and that I could balance their chakras before they arrived for a treatment! I was starting to realise that there were not too many limits to this technique.

Moving beyond a pendulum

On occasion I forgot to bring my pendulum with me, and I could not find anything to use as a substitute, so I started using an 'imaginary pendulum' which I 'held'. My arm made the same muscle movements as before, without the need to suspend a crystal from a thread.

Some people use a pendulum that swings 'in their imagination'. They watch to see how its spin changes in response to their questions. I don't get on very well with that: I never seem to be able to look at the pendulum from the right angle to tell exactly what it is doing!

I tried to move on from this to see if I could dispense with a pendulum altogether, whether real or imaginary. I started 'looking' at someone's chakras by imagining a series of seven circles one above another, and looking at each circle in turn to see whether it was small and closed, or open and large.

I did not trust this to begin with, of course, because I thought 'this is just my imagination... I am making this up', so I went back to my trusted imaginary pendulum, and was amazed to find that the pendulum agreed with my 'imagination'.

Practising visualising chakras

On an update day for my Reiki Masters we practised visualising each other's chakras, and there was a whole variety of presentations. One person saw traffic lights with lights at different intensities.

One saw a string of seven beads. Another could not see anything until she 'peered' over the edge of the chakra, to look down on a lotus flower; some of the flowers had petals that were folded in, others had their petals fully open.

Eventually I moved on from the pendulum, and the imaginary pendulum, and used an imaginary 'mixing desk', rather like you might see in a recording studio: a series of seven vertical 'sliders' with a central point that represents 'balance'. I looked at each chakra slider in turn and if it slid downwards then the chakra was closed or spinning sluggishly, and if it moved upwards then the chakra was spinning too fast.

Now I realise that I do not need to perceive someone's chakras, except out of interest, and certainly I do not need to do anything by way of using Reiki to 'balance' the chakras: Reiki works on the recipient's energy system to achieve more of a state of balance, on all levels, so Reiki works on people's chakras without my having to do anything specific to help, other than by standing by and being a clear channel.

But my experimentation showed me that I was intuitive, that I could trust my intuition, and that I did not need to use 'props': the intuition was there, the intuitive message was there, and the pendulum (or the imaginary pendulum) was just a tool to use to access what was already there within me.

The Japanese connection

The Japanese connection to all this comes in the form of an intuitive 'technique' called "Reiji Ho" which means something like 'indication of the spirit technique'. Details of this method have come to us through Frank Arjava Petter and Hiroshi Doi, and information from Usui's surviving students suggests that this method was probably taught to the Imperial Officers by Usui Sensei.

This method involves allowing the energy to guide your hands to the right places to treat, so rather than following the Western system of 'standard hand positions' you allow Reiki to put your hands in the right place for each person you treat. You are then gearing your treatment to the individual's energy needs, rather than applying a 'rubber stamp' treatment to everyone.

People who I have treated using both approaches have found that intuitive treatments seem to penetrate more deeply, seem more relevant to them and more profound.

Once this technique is mastered then every treatment is different: the hand positions change from one person to another and from one treatment to another with the same client, based on their individual needs. Intuitive treatments are liberating; you just merge with the energy and let it happen!

This was the basis for Usui's original method: letting the energy guide you.

I have described Reiji Ho as a technique, yet in fact there is no method.

The 'technique' involves not doing, not thinking, not trying; in fact it works best if you can simply get your mind out of the way completely.

You feel your connection with the energy, feel the energy flowing through you, and as you do so imagine yourself joining with the energy, merging with the energy, becoming one with the energy... and you simply allow the energy to guide your hands.

What is so exciting for me is that this technique works for almost everyone within a few minutes, so of the 260+ people who have been taught this technique on my 'Original Usui Reiki' update course, more than 95% found that it worked for them almost immediately.

I taught this technique routinely on my Reiki 2 courses and it works incredibly well. The Japanese 'Reiju' empowerments seem to have the effect of giving people greater intuitive potential, so the combination of Reiju and Reiji ho, as well as the energy exercises called Hatsu Rei Ho, work very well together, fitting like the pieces of a simple and elegant jigsaw.

What is also exciting is that if you make it a basic part of your Reiki practice to open yourself to intuition, then you will develop additional intuitive abilities, so moving your hands is only the starting point!

It is liberating and exciting to realise that intuition is there from the start, and that all you have to do to access that inner knowledge is to suspend your disbelief, trust that it will work for you, and have a go.

Don't try hard, don't force it, and don't think about it... just merge with the energy, empty your head, and let it happen!

You can become more intuitive with your Reiki

You are already intuitive

You may not realise it yet, and you may not have too much evidence yet, but you are already intuitive, that is without doubt.

For example, you already know just the right combination of hand positions to use on each person you treat, you already know where the areas of need are, whether they are in front of you or 100 miles away, and you already know just the right amount of time to spend in each hand position.

But at the moment you may not be able to access that intuitive information, the intuition that is already there. Your conscious mind is sitting there like a great big lump, getting in the way and preventing you from accessing what is already there.

Get your mind out of the way

Learning to work intuitively is all about learning to get your conscious mind out of the way, and trusting what comes to you, trusting what you perceive. Working intuitively is all about getting your head out of the way, suspending your disbelief, and allowing it to happen.

To work intuitively you need to not try – it won't work if you *try* – you need to simply be there with the energy, merge with the energy, and let it happen.

So this series of rticles posts is all about helping you to get your mind out of the way, helping you to not try, helping you to merge with the energy, helping you to suspend your disbelief and let it happen.

We will be going through a series of exercises over the coming weeks that you need to practise on other people. This series will not work for you unless you have a group of people available to you to be willing guinea pigs for your intuitive exercises.

- You will learn to cultivate the right state of mind to attract intuitive impressions.
- You will learn to allow your hands to drift with the energy so that "invisible magnets" pull them to the right place to treat.
- You will learn how to use visualisation in different ways to access intuitive knowledge.

A familiar state of mind

Now, the state of mind that you need to cultivate to allow for intuitive working is also the best state of mind to have when practising Reiki, when giving treatments, when carrying out distance healing, when working on yourself.

So these exercises will also help you to develop your ability as a channel and your effectiveness as a practitioner.

We have found that Reiki treatments based on intuitive hand positions do something really special for the recipient, more than if they received treatments based on standard hand positions.

Intuitive treatments seem to allow the energy to penetrate more deeply, to produce effects that are more relevant or more profound.

This makes sense because you are directing the energy into just the right combination of positions for them on that occasion. So from one treatment to another with the same person, you will use different combinations of hand positions, as their energy needs change from one session to another.

Even *you* can become more intuitive!

We have been teaching these intuitive methods for many years now, on live courses and through various Reiki home study courses, and these approaches seem to work for everyone.

The key to working intuitively is to *not* try, and to merge with the energy and to allow it to happen. And the more you get yourself into a lovely empty merged state, the more definite your intuitive impressions will become.

So I wish you an exciting journey with these exercises. You will be following weekly projects, and we explain exactly what you have to do. Follow the instructions; get lots of practice (that's the key to it really), and you will be amazed by what is possible!

I recommend that you keep notes on your experiences as you progress through the course, so you can look back and review your progress.

Develop your Reiki intuition (Part I)

Start by getting the energy flowing

The Reiki attunements give everyone a baseline ability, so you all start off on the same footing.

However, how effective or how 'clear' a channel you are depends on what you do with the energy. It is important to get regular practice, and a good way of getting into a beneficial routine is to spend some time each day carrying out some energy exercises used in Japanese Reiki.

Mikao Usui taught a couple simple Reiki energy exercises to his students when they first started their training with him. The exercises cleanse and purify, start to balance your energy system, and develop the strength of your Reiki channel. They will help to develop your sensitivity to the energy too.

You can read about these exercises in my article "Simple energy exercises to get the energy flowing".

Practising these energy exercises daily will put you in a very good position, energetically-speaking, to practise intuitive working.

Cultivate the right state of mind for Reiki intuition

Here is a solo exercise for you. You can do this by yourself anytime.

Do this exercise for ten minutes each day.

Make yourself comfortable and rest your hands in your lap. Close your eyes. Take a few long deep breaths.

Imagine energy flooding down to you from above, into your crown, and the energy flows down the centre of your body to your Dantien. Feel/imagine the energy building in your Dantien.

A continuous flood of energy keeps pouring through your crown into your Dantien, where it builds.

As the energy floods through you, feel yourself disappearing into the energy and merging with it, imagine yourself becoming one with the energy.

Just be there with the energy, allowing it to flow. No expectations. Just merge with the energy. This is the state that you will be cultivating as you progress through this course.

Over to you

Practise this simple exercise for a week or so.

How does it make you feel? What do you notice?

Develop your Reiki intuition (Part II)

Now we're going to start practising intuitive working with someone else, not just on your own, so you'll need to find some willing volunteers to practise on.

Do this exercise for about five minutes or so for each person you practise on. It doesn't take very long.

Practise on as many people as you can.

Practise compassionate intuition

The recipient sits in a chair or lies on a treatment couch. It doesn't matter which.

Sit near the recipient.

Make yourself comfortable and rest your hands in your lap. Close your eyes.

Take a few long deep breaths.

Imagine energy flooding down to you from above, into your crown, and the energy flows down the centre of your body to your Dantien. Feel/imagine the energy building in your Dantien.

A continuous flood of energy keeps pouring through your crown into your Dantien, where it builds.

As the energy floods through you, feel yourself disappearing into the energy and merging with it, imagine yourself becoming one with the energy. Just be there with the energy, allowing it to flow.

No expectations.

Just merge with the energy for a minute or so.

Now, in your mind, focus your attention on the recipient. Feel yourself merging with them, becoming one with them.

Merge with them for a while.

Take your time with this. There's no rush.

Open your eyes and look at the person with a feeling of gentle compassion, no expectations.

- Do you feel drawn to a particular area or areas of their body?
- Is your attention being pulled towards an area?
- Allow your eyes to drift across their body; do your eyes want to dwell on a particular area?
- Do you feel a physical pull towards a particular area?

Over to you

So, practise this exercise on a variety of people if you can.

See how it becomes more comfortable just letting go and merging with the energy and the recipient.

Develop your Reiki intuition (Part III)

In "Simple energy exercises to get the energy flowing" I walked you through some simple energy exercises that you can carry out every day to clear and cleanse and balance your energy system. In the previous two articles I have also described some exercises that you can carry out on your own, and with a volunteer, to start merging with the energy, and merging with the recipient, opening you up to your intuition.

In this post I am going to describe a Japanese approach to working intuitively, called "Reiji ho", which means something like "indication of the spirit technique".

It's a way of allowing the energy to guide your hands so they drift – rather like being pulled by invisible magnets – to the right place to treat for each person you work on.

How to practise Reiji ho

You will need a willing volunteer for these exercises. Do this exercise for about 10-15 minutes or so for each person you practise on. It doesn't take very long.

Practise on as many people as you can.

The recipient sits in a straight-backed chair and you stand behind them or to one side of them.

Make yourself comfortable and bring your hands into the prayer position. Close your eyes. Take a few long deep breaths.

Imagine energy flooding down to you from above, into your crown, and the energy flows down the centre of your body to your Dantien. Feel/imagine the energy building in your Dantien.

A continuous flood of energy keeps pouring through your crown into your Dantien, where it builds.

As the energy floods through you, feel yourself disappearing into the energy and merging with it, imagine yourself becoming one with the energy. Just be there with the energy, allowing it to flow. No expectations. Just merge with the energy for a minute or so.

Now, in your mind, focus your attention on the recipient. Feel yourself merging with them, becoming one with them. Merge with them for a little while.

Please let me be guided…

Say silently to yourself "please let me be guided"… "please let my hands be guided" … " show me where to treat".

Move your hands so that they are hovering near the recipient's head in a neutral, comfortable position. Your hands and arms are loose, there is no resistance; your hands will drift smoothly and easily.

Imagine the energy is flooding through you: into your crown, through your arms and out of your hands. Feel yourself disappearing into the energy, merging with the energy, becoming one with the energy... and allow your hands to drift.

There is no resistance; your hands will drift and glide smoothly and easily.

Allow your hands to drift

As you do this you may notice a gentle or subtle pull on your hands.

Allow them to drift until they come to rest. You may now have a feeling that your hands are in the 'right' place, and you may feel a lot of energy flowing through your hands. Allow the energy to flow for a minute.

Now bring your hands back to your 'start' position (whatever position that was) and repeat the process. You are practising allowing your hands to drift with the energy; you are not practising treating someone at the moment.

Keep on moving your hands back into the start position, and allow them to drift to where they want to go.

Some things to notice

- Sometimes both hands will drift and come to a stop, and on other occasions only one hand will move.
- Sometimes a hand will drift further away from the body, or move closer to the body. In the latter case do look to see where your hand is going!
- Sometimes a hand will not come to rest, but will keep moving in an interesting 'energy dance'. Just go with

271

the flow and accept what happens as the right thing for the recipient on that occasion.

In practice, wherever your hands come to rest, you would rest your hands on the person to treat, obviously depending on the part of the body your hands are hovering over: some areas should be treated with the hands hovering above the body, not resting on the surface, for the sake of propriety.

Over to you

Practise the Reiji ho method with as many people as you can get your hands on, and see what you notice.

What happens? Where do your hands drift?

Remember that the key to success with this intuitive technique is to give up and stop trying: you can't force this.

Develop your Reiki intuition (Part IV)

In this post I am going to talk about using Reiji ho with a recipient who is resting on a treatment table in front of you, and how you can use Reiji ho in practice when you treat people, when you carry out full treatments.

How to start your Reiji ho

Do this exercise for about 15 minutes or so for each person you practise on. It doesn't take very long.

Practise on as many people as you can.

The recipient lies on a treatment couch and you stand beside them.

Make yourself comfortable and bring your hands into the prayer position. Close your eyes. Take a few long deep breaths. Imagine energy flooding down to you from above, into your crown, and the energy flows down the centre of your body to your Dantien. Feel/imagine the energy building in your Dantien.

A continuous flood of energy keeps pouring through your crown into your Dantien, where it builds.

As the energy floods through you, feel yourself disappearing into the energy and merging with it, imagine yourself becoming one with the energy. Just be there with the energy, allowing it to flow. No expectations. Just merge with the energy for a minute or so.

Now, in your mind, focus your attention on the recipient. Feel yourself merging with them, becoming one with them.

Merge with them for a little while.

Say silently to yourself "please let me be guided"… "please let my hands be guided" … " show me where to treat".

Hover your hands in neutral

Move your hands so that they are hovering over the recipient's torso in a neutral, comfortable position

Your hands and arms are loose, there is no resistance; your hands will drift smoothly and easily.

Imagine the energy is flooding through you: into your crown, through your arms and out of your hands.

Feel yourself disappearing into the energy, merging with the energy, becoming one with the energy… and allow your hands to drift.

There is no resistance; your hands will drift and glide smoothly and easily.

Allow your hands to drift

As you do this you may notice a gentle or subtle pull on your hands. Allow them to drift until they come to rest. You may now have a feeling that your hands are in the 'right' place, and you may feel a lot of energy flowing through your hands.

Allow the energy to flow for a minute.

Now bring your hands back to your 'start' position (whatever position that was) and repeat the process. You are practising allowing your hands to drift with the energy; you are not practising treating someone at the moment.

Keep on moving your hands back into the start position, and allow them to drift to where they want to go.

Now move to another part of the body, so you are standing next to the hips, or the knees, and repeat the exercise, each time seeing where your hands want to drift, allowing them to come to rest if they want to, and repeating the process to see if they drift to the same area each time.

Some things to notice

- Sometimes both hands will drift and come to a stop, and on other occasions only one hand will move.
- Sometimes a hand will drift further away from the body, or move closer to the body. In the latter case do look to see where your hand is going!
- Sometimes a hand will not come to rest, but will keep moving in an interesting 'energy dance'. Just go with the flow and accept what happens as the right thing for the recipient on that occasion.

In practice, wherever your hands come to rest, you would rest your hands on the person to treat, obviously depending on the part of the body your hands are hovering over: some areas should be treated with the hands hovering above the body, not resting on the surface, for the sake of propriety.

When your hands come to rest you usually find that there is a lot of energy coming through. This makes sense because you have just put your hands in just the right combination of positions for that person on that occasion.

After a while you will notice that the flow of energy subsides, and you know that it is ok to move on to the next combination of hand positions. If you move your hands away too soon you will simply be guided back to those positions to treat some more!

In practice you will find that you end up with fewer hand positions than you used when following your 'standard' hand positions.

In practice I always treat someone's shoulders for about 10 minutes when I start a treatment.

Then I move on to use Reiji ho on the head. Usually I end up with 'non-symmetrical' hand positions. Then after say 25 minutes I move on to the torso and let the energy guide me there, and I stay in each hand position until I feel that it is right to move on.

Over to you

Practise the method I have described on as many people as you can. What you are doing is practising and getting used to 'giving up and not trying', just merging with the energy and letting it happen. That's the key to success with Reiji ho.

The Importance of Intent

A wise friend of mine once said to me that "where thought goes, energy flows" and I think that this principle applies very well to Reiki.

Some of us have been taught in quite a rigid way, learning that we must always follow a particular prescription to achieve a desired effect, whether this be a set form of words, a collection of symbols, or a complicated ritual. That's fine: we can choose to do that if we like, but I believe that underlying our form of words, our rituals and our symbols is an important and powerful driving force: our intention.

I believe that we can move beyond the details, the constructed systems, to access that simple, profound and powerful controlling force.

Whatever we do, when we do Reiki, we control the energy using our intention.

Reiki through breathing and staring

Many people are now experimenting with sending Reiki using their eyes and their breath, based on the two Japanese techniques 'Gyoshi Ho' and 'Koki Ho'. Now I do not believe that Reiki necessarily comes out of your eyeballs when you use the 'eye' technique, like Clark Kent raising his glasses to send laser beams out of his eyes. But I do think that you have created a little visualisation that sends the energy in a particular way.

When you imagine that Reiki passes from your eyes, the energy is focused in a way that picks up on some of the connotations of staring: the energy is received in a piercing, localised, penetrating, or 'focused' way.

Send using your breath and the energy is sent in more of a superficial 'billowing' form.

You have made the energy go to the other person's body. You have intended that, and it has happened. You visualised to achieve this, but that is just a convenient way of focusing your intent, and it is your intent that is the important thing here, not the details of the ritual that you use to control the energy.

We don't need big rituals

You may choose to carry out a detailed ritual in order to perform distant healing, you may use a set form of words, a symbol, more symbols, you may make a detailed visualisation, but you are still focusing your intent and the details of the ritual don't matter.

If you feel comfortable with detailed ritual - 'High Church' - then fine, that works for you; stick with that. But I think we need to realise that we can remove the strait jacket, we can let the ritual go if we want to and still achieve the desired effect, and that is still Reiki.

We can experiment: sit a Reiki friend the other side of the room and send Reiki to their forehead, or their shoulder. Don't beam it, don't do distant healing, don't use your eyes or your hands: sit on your hands, close your eyes and just *make* the energy go where you want. It will follow your thoughts.

When you are thinking nice warm thoughts about another person then dzzzzt, the energy has followed your thoughts, your focus, and you have just sent distant healing to them.

When we self-treat we can move the energy through our bodies using our mind, using our intention. If you can't contort yourself and get your hands to rest on the part that you want to treat, just imagine that your hands are resting on the area that you want to treat, and the energy will be there.

If you have backache, and you were lying on your bed with your hands resting on your abdomen, you could imagine - visualise - that the energy was flowing from your hands to your back, and the energy would go there.

You can even 'cut out the middle man': draw down the energy through your crown and imagine it passing through your body to the affected area. The energy will go there.

Moving beyond symbols

The symbols, too, are a visual focus that connects us to a particular aspect of the energy that is already within us. Usui introduced symbols late on in Reiki's history for the benefit of the Imperial Officers who trained with him. They are the foundation of Western Reiki, though not of the 'original' form of Reiki that Usui Sensei taught to most of his students.

We can go beyond the symbols too if we feel that we want to, once we have experienced the distinctive flavours, the distinctive energies, of the Reiki symbols. Unfortunately the

Western way does not tend to give us this opportunity, but the potential is there.

What lies behind each symbol is a distinctive, characteristic energy, and with practice we can move the symbol to one side and access the energies direct if we choose, and that is still Reiki.

We can limit our practice of Reiki with our belief. If we believe that something is not possible, or not 'correct', then we are shooting ourselves in the foot before we even begin.

If we believe that something is not possible then we will not try, we will not maximise our potential, and our Reiki is diminished as a result.

If we can raise our horizons, suspend our disbelief, and simply try things, then we will be amazed by what is possible, and how simple things can be.

"Where thought goes, energy flows."

Scanning at a distance

Using props

In "How to send Reiki distant healing (Part IV)" I spoke about different 'props' that you can use when sending distant healing: sending Reiki into a teddy bear, or a pillow, or even into your upper leg.

All these props serve to represent the recipient's body, helping you to focus your attention on the recipient and direct the energy into a particular part of their body at a distance. You are bolstering your intent by using the prop to make your intention 'concrete'.

But in the same way that you are using the intermediate of the teddy bear, say, to help 'transmit' the energy, you can also receive information from the recipient about where the energy wants to go in greatest amounts, and we can do this by 'scanning' the teddy bear (or pillow).

Scanning a prop

Scanning, when used on a client on a treatment table in front of you, is a method where you hover your hand(s) over their body, a few inches away, and drift your hands from one place to another, paying attention to the sensations of heat, pulsing, fizzing, tingling, heaviness etc in your hands, by way of finding those areas that are drawing most energy, so that you can spend longer treating those areas.

Your hands can then guide you in terms of how long you treat in a particular area since you will notice that, after a while, the flow of energy subsides and you can then move on to another hand position.

And we can scan the teddy bear of pillow, who represents the recipient, and we can hover our hands, drifting our hand from one place to another, noticing the flow of energy through our hand into the prop, into the recipient.

An area of great need in the recipient will show itself by a more intense flow of energy into a particular part of the prop.

Just like in a live Reiki treatment, when you find an area on the prop that is drawing a lot of energy then you can treat that area for longer, until the flow of energy subsides.

So the distant connection to the recipient works two ways: as a way of directing Reiki to them, and also as a way of receiving information about where the energy needs to go.

Over to you

If you haven't experimented with this sort of thing before, why not have a go

Remote Treatments

When is a distant healing session not a distant healing session? ... When it is a remote treatment!

What is a remote treatment? Well that is what I hope to describe in this article, and I also want to talk a little bit about 'removing the barriers' when you treat someone, going freestyle; I will outline some of the things that are possible when you simply suspend your disbelief, and try things out to see what's possible.

Now distant healing is based on the idea of making a long-distance 'connection' with the recipient, maybe by using a symbol, maybe by using a sacred sound, or maybe simply when you still your mind and you find that space where you are 'at one', merging with the other person.

"Connection" is a state of mind

Your 'connection' to the recipient is a state of mind, a matter of your intention, and the details of the ritual that you use are not important.

Some Reiki people are taught that they need to keep at least one hand on the recipient at all times when they carry out hands-on treatments - otherwise they'll 'lose the connection' - but of course you are 'connected' to the recipient just as much when your hands are hovering away from the body.

Your 'connection' does not depend on the physical proximity of your hands to someone's body. You are connected with your intention, when you are still and focused, you are connected as soon as you direct your attention towards the recipient.

But let's get back to distant healing. In practice this tends to be carried out for 10-15 minutes at a time over a number of consecutive days, and we send the energy to the person for their highest good, in a 'general' way, not directing the energy to a particular area.

But since our 'connection' to the person is a state of mind, we could maintain that 'distant' connection for a prolonged period if we wanted, and we could direct the energy with our intention to different specific parts of the recipient's body, in the same way that when we treat someone we direct the energy with our hands to specific areas of the body.

And since with Reiki the energy follows our thoughts, it follows our focus; we can direct the energy using visualisation, which is a convenient shortcut to focus our intent.

Carrying out a remote treatment

We can if we like carry out a "remote treatment', where we maintain our connection to the recipient for maybe 30-40 minutes and direct the energy into the recipient's body by using imaginary hand positions. The energy will enter the recipient's body in the areas we imagine/intend.

What hand positions should we use? Well we could go through a set of 'standard' hand positions, but we should learn to move beyond that as soon as we can: far better would be to use our intuition, and a good way of working out where our hands should go is to use the Japanese intuitive 'technique' called "Reiji Ho".

"Reiji ho" is basically a way of getting your head out of the way, merging with the energy and allowing your hands to move, rather like having your hands moved by invisible magnets. Just like dowsing or automatic writing, Reiji Ho allows us to tap in to subconscious knowledge, and that knowledge is expressed through muscle movements. We already know the best places to put our hands, but quite often our mind gets in the way and stops us from getting to that deep knowing. Reiji helps to get our head out of the way for us.

So once you are connected to the other person in your mind, you can imagine them lying down on a treatment couch and visualise imaginary hands resting on or hovering over them. In your mind's eye, 'look' at your hands and see where they want to drift. They will drift in your mind's eye; be neutral, simply interested to see where they come to rest. When they come to rest, direct Reiki into your subject in those areas using intent; imagine energy flooding through those imaginary hands into the recipient's body.

The energy will enter the recipient's body in the places that you imagine.

Deciding how long to stay in a hand position

How long should you keep your hands in a particular position? Maybe you have a feeling that you ought to move on to a different position, but you're not sure whether you should yet. Here's a way to see if you should move on: in your mind's eye, pull one of your imaginary hands away from the place where it was resting; if it wants to slip back to that place again, rather like it was attached by an elastic band, then you can stay there for longer, directing the energy into the body in that position until you feel that the imaginary hand will drift away easily.

This visualisation can be used when you are doing hands-on treatments too, to let you know whether it's ok to move on to the next hand position.

Then 'see' where your imaginary hands want to drift next, and direct energy into your 'remote treatment' recipient using your visualisation or intent. This is a lovely way to work, because you have to really merge with the energy, to become one with the energy, to do this.

In fact you can even 'scan' the recipient at a distance if you want. Hover one hand in mid-air, palm down, and in your mind's eye imagine your hand drift over the recipient's body. Notice the areas where there seems to be a lot of energy flowing in your hand.

Try it. It works!

So why don't you try an experiment: get a willing victim to lie down at a prearranged time for, say, 45 minutes. Connect to them in your head, using your intent, let the energy guide your imaginary hands, direct the energy using visualisation (using intent) and see what you perceive.

Go with the flow. See what they notice.

Suspend your disbelief and see what happens!

Feng Shui your Reiki

Many of you will be familiar with Feng Shui, the Oriental art of placement, where you arrange your living environment to allow smooth flow of chi through your home, eliminating areas where chi will stagnate, and slowing down the speed of fast-rushing chi.

So what has that to do with Reiki? Well they both deal with chi, but what I am really thinking of is applying the basic principles of Feng Shui to our practice of Reiki. This may seem a little strange, but please bear with me...

Get rid of your clutter

The basic principle of Feng Shui, the first thing you have to do before you do anything else, is to get rid of your clutter, because a cluttered environment leads to a cluttered life. Only once you have rid yourself of your unnecessary bits and pieces should you move in to apply the other more specific principles of placement.

So could we de-clutter our practice of Reiki, what would that be like, and how could we achieve that? Is our Reiki cluttered now? How could we pare it down to the essentials and leave the unnecessary stuff behind?

We do seem to have a tendency in the West to make things endlessly complicated, almost on the basis that if it's more complicated then it's better. We like to introduce rules and regulations and restrictions and dogma, maybe because rules make us feel supported and safe, or maybe because we just can't leave a simple thing alone!

Yet the system that Usui Sensei taught to his surviving students wasn't complicated. It wasn't cluttered. It was simple and elegant and profound, and I think that we've drifted away from that in many ways.

We've introduced rules and restrictions and dogma into many aspects of Reiki practice: connecting to the energy, treating someone, hand positions, distant healing methods, situations where you 'should not treat'. This is all clutter and we can do without it.

Freeing ourselves from this burden of technique and method and limitation would be a great and beneficial clear-out. We don't need it. It holds us back.

Let's look at a few examples of unnecessary clutter...

A 15-stage connection ritual!

A while ago I was contacted by a poor girl who had been taught that she needed to go through a fifteen-stage ritual in order to 'connect' to Reiki. She and the other students on the course were quite worried, obviously concerned that if they didn't get all the stages right then the energy wouldn't come through properly and their treatments would be ineffective.

Naturally they wanted to do the very best they could for the people they were working on, and they were focusing hard on getting all the necessary stages right.

Yet 'connection' with Reiki is simply a state of mind; you connect when you intend to connect. Some people will hold their hands in a particular position (hands above them with palms uppermost to the sky, hands to the sides with palms face up, hands in the prayer position, hands in their lap with palms up, hands folded over the Dantien). Maybe they will say a set form of words, but all these are optional. Bring the energy through your crown to your Dantien and bathe in the light, flood the energy through your body, be still; you are connected when you intend to be. It is a matter of focus, a matter of where your attention lies.

Keep at least one hand on someone at all times?

Some people are taught that they must always keep one of their hands in contact with the recipient when they treat, based on the idea that if you take both hands off then you have lost your connection to the recipient and the energy will not flow properly.

But your connection to the recipient is a state of mind too: you focus your attention on them, you merge with them and become one with them, and that is sufficient no matter what you are doing with your hands.

In fact your treatment starts as soon as you are standing by the table with your attention directed towards the person. Your treatment has already started when you are scanning, or feeling the energy field. Reiki works just as well when you have your hands off the body, though Reiki is basically practised as a hands-on method.

Following standard hand positions in all circumstances

Some Reiki people are taught rigid 'standard' hand positions that have to be used every time you treat, and there is the view that if you are not using 'the' hand positions then you haven't been taught properly. Some even have a rigid time limit that has to be followed, so you can only keep your hands in each position for so many minutes... you can buy Reiki CDs which make a little 'ping' sound every three minutes (or whatever), and everyone changes hand positions like a robot.

Yet what if your hands are going like crazy, what if there energy needs to flood into a particular area for a long time and you need to keep your hands there for 5 minutes or 10 minutes or 15 minutes?

The answer would seem to be that you follow the system rigidly and ignore your hands.

How sad.

Moving beyond standard hand positions

Of course, standard hand positions are useful when you first learn Reiki: it's reassuring to have some sort of system to follow. But we can move beyond those standard hand positions in a couple of ways.

When we 'scan' the body we night discover areas that are drawing lots of Reiki, but they aren't covered by the 'standard' hand positions... we can alter our hand positions accordingly, or add extra positions, to make sure we're directing the energy into the areas that are drawing the most Reiki.

We can use intuition, too, to control our hand positioning, and this has great benefits for the recipient because we are directing the energy into just the right combination of positions for each person we are working on. We might feel inexplicably 'drawn' to a particular area, we might just 'know' that we ought to be treating a particular area, or we might be practicing "Reiji Ho" from Japan, where our hands are drawn by 'invisible magnets' to the right areas to treat. Again we are leaving the rigid standard positions to one side and going with the flow.

That was Usui's way: there were no real standard positions. You simply put your hands where they wanted to go.

Ditching distant healing rules and regulations

Distant healing is another area where lots of rules and regulations have crept in over time. Some people are taught quite complicated rituals that they have to carry out when they perform distant healing, with a set form of words that 'have' to be used in a particular way, and with various required visualisations.

Yet the bare bones of distant healing are to know where the energy is to go – to set a firm intent – to use the distant healing symbol maybe, and to merge with the recipient, allowing the energy to flow. Anything beyond that is optional.

People have different styles: some like to actively visualise and develop a detailed ritual, and that's fine, but it's not actually necessary. Others like to keep it simple, and that works just as well. Even the use of the distant healing symbol is optional, though it does help us to focus on merging with the recipient, a way of experiencing 'oneness' with the person you're sending the energy to.

Distant healing is perfectly possible at First Degree level, too: it's simple a matter of intent, of focusing your attention in a particular way. The energy follows your thoughts, it follows your focus.

Ditch Reiki "contraindications"

The final area where we could give our Reiki a big 'clear out' is in the rules and restrictions that can control who we should and should not treat. Some people are given a long list of 'contraindications': situations where you should not give Reiki because it might be dangerous.

Some contraindications that I have come across include: pregnant women, babies, people with pacemakers, diabetics*, people undergoing an anaesthetic, people wearing contact lenses, people with cancer, people suffering from stress, people with broken bones, people taking homoeopathic remedies, people undergoing chemotherapy, people with a torn muscle.

There will be many more examples taught in different lineages. These restrictions are nonsense, they have no basis: there is no proper evidence – even anecdotes – to back up the restrictions that are taught in some lineages. Reiki is safe, the person's body draws it to the right areas to treat, and Reiki is seen as divinely inspired, intelligent, it is seen as pure unconditional love. That view hardly sits too well with the suggestion that you can hurt someone using Reiki.

We think too much, we worry too much, and we create problems where there are none.

So a practice of Reiki that follows the first principle of Feng Shui will be a simple practice, free from rules, restrictions and self-imposed limitations. Feng Shui'd Reiki will be free from dogma, and free from rituals that you 'must' follow for Reiki to work effectively.

It will be a practice that is based on simple intent and intuition, where you merge with the recipient, where you become one with them, and where you let the energy guide you. Let's get rid of all that clutter and free up our practice, and just let the energy flow.

[* There is some anecdotal evidence that some diabetics may experience a short term alteration in blood sugar levels following a Reiki treatment. They should be made aware of this possibility and monitor their sugar levels accordingly. However, this does not mean that you should not treat diabetics using Reiki, as is suggested in some quarters. It just means that diabetics should keep an eye on their blood sugar levels following a Reiki treatment or a course of Reiki treatments. They should be checking their blood sugar levels routinely in any case.]

Beware Reiki "know-it-alls"

A Reiki practitioner contacted me the other day to ask my advice about something. They had treated a new Reiki client, who had been to see other Reiki practitioners in the past, and the client wanted to know what the practitioner had picked up, meaning that the client wanted the Reiki practitioner to tell her about physical problems she had: to diagnose what was wrong with the client.

The client commented that previous Reiki practitioners they had seen had told them that they had a problem with a particular part of their body (maybe an organ).

This made the practitioner feel very uncomfortable because she did not feel qualified to do something like that, to diagnose.

And that is the sensible response.

Because for Reiki practitioners to try and diagnose is outrageous behaviour:

- Reiki practitioners cannot diagnose.
- Reiki practitioners are not qualified to diagnose.
- Reiki is not a system that is set up to diagnose.

Doctors diagnose. We don't.

The fact that there might be a lot of energy going into a particular part of the body does not mean that there is a physical problem with the bit of the body your hand is resting on, because Reiki works on lots of levels: it deals with unhelpful thoughts, it helps with unbalanced or repressed emotions and it deals with the physical level too.

Reiki will flow into a person to deal with historical stuff that has still left a trace on some level and which needs to be restored or balanced in some way, and it will also deal with new stuff that's 'on the boil' and may never manifest itself as an actual physical problem.

Reiki will work on the spiritual level too, giving the client what they need on many levels.

In Traditional Chinese Medicine (TCM) thoughts and emotions are believed to reside in particular organs, for example the liver energy relates to the emotion of anger, the kidney relates to fear and the lung relates to grief. Problems with mental states like planning and decision-making, organising your thoughts, bringing plans to fruition, and the like, reside in different organs of the body.

So do you really know what they energy is dealing with when it flows into your client?

We don't diagnose. And how arrogant to believe that we can.

Some Reiki practitioners will tell a client that they have 'dark energy' in their liver. I have heard of people doing that! Dark energy?? How is that even a helpful concept to have?

Saying such a thing imposes the practitioner's worldview on their client and will seriously freak them out. If you have dark energy in your body, you will want to know how to get rid of it, and get rid of it now!

Presumably only the all-knowing, all-powerful Reiki practitioner, trained in the esoteric arts, can sort it out for them.

What can I safely say?

So, what we can say that is useful and honouring when a client asks what we noticed or 'picked up on'?

We can say something like this: "I noticed quite a lot of energy going into this area of the body.

Often a client will say, "oh, that's because of…" and the client will be reassured that you 'picked up on' some condition or problem or injury that they knew about and you didn't.

It reassures them that Reiki is actually going where it is needed.

Let's add some Clairvoyance, shall we?

It is clear that learning Reiki, and practising Reiki, does seem to enhance the psychic or clairvoyant ability in some people.

But should we start blurting out every image and impression that comes into our heads when we treat someone? No, we should not.

Your client came for a Reiki treatment, not a clairvoyant consultation. Making such comments unsolicited is intrusive and may well be unhelpful and unwelcome.

Especially to begin with, are you really sure what you are imagining is not just a random thought, as your mind wanders?

I advise caution.

For Masters

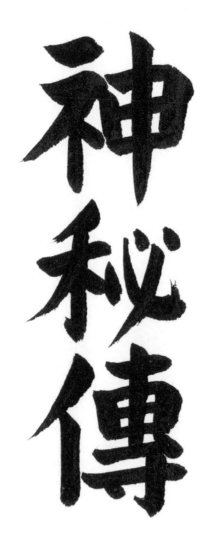

Do attunements actually work?

A bit of a cheeky question!

I thought this title might attract some attention!

There are some silly people in the world of Reiki who are squitting about Reiju empowerments and suggesting that they don't do anything, so I thought I would turn the tables slightly by posing the question, "what do attunements do, anyway?"

The received wisdom that comes through the general Western approach to Reiki is that attunements "attune" you, in that they connect you to an energy source that you weren't connected to before, opening you up to something that wasn't part of your world before the rituals took place.

But is that really what it's all about?

I don't believe so.

Connected to something new and different?

I'm going to put to one side for the moment that fact that Usui Sensei didn't use or teach attunements – he never attuned anyone to anything – and let's think about this idea that an attunement connects you to something different, something new, a new energy source.

How can that be?

How can there be something so fundamental that we aren't already part of?

If we think about the Buddhist origins of Reiki, one of the principles of Buddhism is that reality is illusion: the idea of us being separate individuals, distinct from other people, is illusion; the true reality is that of oneness... we are not separate. Mikao Usui was a Buddhist. Mainly, he taught people who were Buddhists or followers of Shinto.

Would he have established an energetic system, when his whole worldview was based on the idea of oneness, that was based on the idea of connecting you to something different, separate and distinct from you, when this went against everything he believed in?

I don't think so.

So, for me, attunements don't hook you up to a new energy source that you didn't have access to before. What they do is to 'flag up' to you something that has always been there as a part of you, ready to use. Attunements are a way of helping you to notice something that has always been there but which has been out of your awareness and thus not easily accessible to you.

I hope a couple of metaphors will help here...

"The high-pitched sound"

Imagine that you walk into your friend's lounge and they say to you, "can you hear that high-pitched noise?". You listen and you can't hear anything. They say, "no, listen, it's there".

You try again and, by altering the way that you are focusing your attention, perhaps by tilting your head, by being aware of sounds that aren't of the usual frequencies, you become able to hear the sound that was there all the time, but to begin with you were unable to hear it.

Your friend 'made the introductions' between your awareness and something that you did not have access to before.

A NLP metaphor

One of the principles of NLP (Neuro Linguistic Programming) is that in order for us to be able to function, our subconscious minds are obliged to take the millions of bits of information that come in through our senses every second, and ditch most of them by using 'filters' that distort, delete and generalise what is coming through to us.

Without this we'd never move; we don't have the processing power to deal with all the inputs that come to us.

One of the ways that we filter thing is based on what we have been focusing our attention on. Many people will have noticed that if they are thinking of buying a particular brand of car, they suddenly start to notice that car everywhere they go. Examples of that car have always been around with that sort of frequency but they were previously unimportant to us and so 'deleted' from our conscious awareness.

A new 'filter' has been set up that says, "notice this type of car" and our unconscious mind brings into our awareness something that has always been there but which is now within our awareness.

Attunements do this too, setting up a new 'filter' that brings to our attention something that has always been there, an integral part of you, but hidden behind a veil.

Click your fingers to attract someone's attention

So rather like someone who shouts to you, "Hey", clicks their fingers a few times, saying, "look at this, here, look, notice this, feel this", attunements help to bring into our awareness something that has always been there.

And once you are able to notice those high-pitched sounds, for example, you can always 'tune into' them. As with Reiki, once you've been given the knack of focusing on and becoming aware of what is there, you can always do it.

Do attunements actually work?

Well the answer is both yes and no.

They don't connect you to something new and different and separate from you, because there is no such thing, though they do allow you access to 'the energy' which has always been there with you.

And that's all you need.

Become a super power Reiki Master in just 48 hours? What a joke!

Roll up, roll up!

Roll up, roll up, and get your Reiki Mastership here. No effort involved. Just visit this page, look at this, download this and pay your money. All done online.

You are now a super-power Reiki Master with amazing abilities, more than a mere mortal. You have your Reiki Master cape, your Reiki Master all-seeing eye, super-power intuition and phenomenal super power energy.

Really?

Is that what we think Reiki Mastery is all about? Is it a title that you earn by flipping a switch, paying by PayPal, going on a course for a couple of days and there you have it – you're a **MASTER**.

Nothing more to do.

I don't think that's what Reiki Mastery is all about

It's not an event, it's a state of mind, it's a form of commitment, it's a journey.

It's about how you behave and how you conduct yourself.

In Usui Sensei's original system, Shinpiden level was a path to 'satori', a flash of insight that changes something in a fundamental way (something that comes through a long period of meditation, something that you work at by getting rid of your 'baggage').

The highest level of Reiki development was left open-ended, a lifelong journey, for you to progress as far as you could progress, through your own efforts.

In a hundred years that has morphed in some quarters into something that you can get in a leisurely afternoon surfing the Internet.

I prefer to use the term 'Reiki teacher' rather than 'Reiki Master' because the phrase 'Reiki Teacher' describes perfectly what most people at that level do, without all the added connotations of superhuman abilities.

When you become a Reiki Master, you start on the bottom rung!

For me, Reiki mastery begins when you have completed your RMT course, and you are on the bottom rung.

I know that some RMT courses are basically just about learning how to attune people, but they're not all like that and many courses give you tools that you can use to develop yourself further, and your Reiki mastery is a journey of dedication and commitment, where you work on yourself long-term; it's about self development, personal development, it's about embracing mindfulness and embodying the precepts in your daily life, not seeking perfection but seeking to develop further over time.

So Reiki mastery is about how you commit yourself to work on yourself long-term, it's about how you relate to other people in your daily life, how you relate to your students, it's about the way that you 'sit' with the energy, it's about your humility and your compassion and your forgiveness, and your contentment in the moment.

It's not a piece of paper.

What comes to mind is the probably apocryphal story where, when attaining their martial arts black belts, students are told that, finally, they have reached the stage of being a beginner. It all starts there.

So next time you see one of those adverts telling you that you can become a super-power Reiki Master online just like that [clicks fingers], think about what Reiki Mastery really means and whether what you are being offered by these people is actually worth obtaining.

Over to you

So what do you think of these "become a Reiki Master overnight" or "train at all three Reiki levels in a weekend" courses?

The founder of Western Reiki did distant attunements!

A very awkward discovery

As we know, Western-style Reiki has drawn to itself a lot of dogma, rigidity and blinkered-thinking, and nowhere is this more prevalent than in the area of distant attunements.

As far as many Reiki teachers and societies are concerned, teaching Reiki to someone who isn't sitting in front of you is tantamount to heresy and we are all expected to believe that distant attunements do not work.

In fact, if I recall this correctly, one of the requirements of the UK Reiki Council's core curriculum is that the student, to be properly taught Reiki, has to believe that attunements must carried out face to face, so we even have Reiki thought-police at large in the world!

This is nonsense, of course, and it takes quite some mental gymnastics to believe both that Reiki can be sent from one side of the planet to the other just by thinking about it (à la distant healing) while maintaining that you can only be initiated into Reiki by being corraled in the same room as your teacher for some close-quarters mystical hand-waving.

Mrs Takata has put the cat amongst the pigeons!

But new evidence has just come to light which shows that Mrs Hawayo Takata, the lady responsible for teaching Dr Hayashi's version of Reiki in the Western world, the source of Western Reiki, actually gave a distant attunement and taught someone remotely, in fact 'over the telephone'.

The research was carried out by Robert Fueston, who was examining archive material at the David M. Rubenstein Rare Book & Manuscript Library at Duke University. You can read a fuller report on this by visiting Pamela Miles's Reiki website.

This is very important.

Hawayo Takata was *the* source of Reiki in the West and until very recently all Reiki practitioners and Masters will have had Mrs T sitting there in their lineage. In many quarters, Mrs Takata's approach and her teachings are almost sacrosanct and underpin the approach of the Reiki Alliance, for example, or the Reiki Association in the UK.

And it will be these more 'traditional' organisations who will be dead against any sort of distant teaching of Reiki.

But now we know that distant teaching, and distant initiations, were right there from the very beginning.

Dangerous knowledge?

I was a little disappointed when reading the report of Robert Fueston's endeavours that he "felt conflicted about releasing this information, lest it be taken as a precedent to justify remote teaching" and he goes on to try and limit the application of distant teaching, saying that Mrs Takata "only used remote initiations when it seemed absolutely necessary" and "this way of teaching was the exception rather than the norm."

What are people afraid of?

Either it works or it doesn't!

And if it works, it doesn't have to be limited to 'emergencies' only.

My experience of teaching at a distance

Distant attunements and distance Reiki training work.

I have taught Reiki to students all over the world. I have taught 500+ people in 28 countries, in fact, from USA to UAE, from the Netherlands to Netherlands Antilles, from Norway to Taiwan.

All my students have been initiated at a distance and have followed courses that gave them far more practical, hands-on experience of using Reiki on themselves and other people than is possible on any sort of live course.

When carried properly, distant Reiki courses are just as good as live training, with the distinct advantage that you can have the one-to-one attention of your teacher over an extended period and you can take your time, getting all the hands-on practice that you need and only moving on when you feel comfortable with what you have learned.

But don't take my word for it! If you visit the Reiki Evolution and find your way to the Reiki home study courses pages, you will find endless testimonials from people who have learned Reiki at a distance and become confident and experienced practitioners.

Attunements, empowerments & the Reiki contact lens scandal!

Some people have weird ideas, even for Reiki!

In this article I would like to talk a bit about **attunements and empowerments** used in Reiki, explaining the similarities and differences between these rituals.

I was prompted to write this article after reading a message posted to an Internet discussion group a while ago, on the subject of **Reiju empowerments**. The message contained such a lot of misinformation and distortions that one could have concluded that it was posted mischievously, or maliciously, for 'political' reasons.

Just the other day I smiled broadly because I came across an item on a web page which was trying to argue that the empowerments used by Mikao Usui were ineffective in connecting people to Reiki!

Very strange.

In any case, hopefully I can clear up some confusion or misunderstandings that people might have about attunements and empowerments, and this article should be of interest to people at all Reiki levels.

As for the contact lenses, you can find out about them towards the end of this article!

Connection rituals

No matter what sort of Reiki course you choose to follow, wherever you are in the world, you are likely to go through a ritual or a series of rituals which can be seen as a way of 'connecting' you to Reiki, a way of hooking you up to something that you were previously not connected to.

That is a common way that such rituals are viewed: a way of 'attuning' you to something that you were not attuned to before, a way of plugging you into a new source of energy that was not available to you before.

But perhaps it is more useful to say that an empowerment, or an attunement, is a 'ritual permission', a permission to recognise something that is within, something that has always been there.

The effect of the connection ritual is to allow you to channel energy for your own benefit, and for other people's benefit, in a way that was not possible for you before you went through the ritual with your Reiki teacher.

Most people in the world of Reiki have been 'connected' using an "attunement" ritual, a version of the ritual that Mrs Takata was using, and while increasing numbers are now being connected using an "empowerment", for the foreseeable future those attuned will always outnumber those empowered: most Reiki teachers attune, only a minority empower.

What are Reiki "attunements"

Until approximately 1999, everyone within the world of Reiki will have been 'attuned' using some sort of variation of the connection ritual that Hawayo Takata taught to the Masters that she initiated in the 1970s.

Since the '70s Reiki has spread throughout the world and the attunement rituals used have evolved and changed as they have been passed from one teacher to another down the line.

Some attunements are now quite complicated affairs, with many, many stages, while others are fairly simple, though there are some common themes that seem to run through most methods, for example the placing of the Reiki symbols into different parts of the student's body (head and hands for example), tapping, blowing, affirming, visualising.

So there is not one standard attunement ritual used in the world of Reiki: there are endless variations, some quite contradictory to each other; if one method works in terms of the 'theory' behind it then a very different method does not make 'sense' and simply cannot work, and yet all methods do seem to work perfectly well.

Some people insist that there have to be four attunements for Reiki First Degree, which is a big historical misunderstanding that I will not go into now, while others use three, or two, or even one attunement on their courses.

All these approaches work.

Mikao Usui did not 'attune' people

It should be stated that Mikao Usui did not give people attunements, he did not attune anyone to any symbols, and he did not teach attunements. Attunements were not part of the system that Usui taught: he used empowerments instead.

Usui taught empowerments to his Master students, and this was not done early on in their Master training – passing on the Reiki ability to others was only taught towards the end of the Master student's formal training with Usui Sensei.

Now, the Imperial Officers who trained with Usui had not trained with him for long enough to have reached the level where they would have been taught to empower others, so where did the attunements used on most Reiki courses come from? Interestingly, it seems that after Usui's untimely death the Imperial Officers put together a ritual that replicated the feelings or the experiences that they had when being empowered by Usui.

Dr Hayashi passed on such a ritual to Mrs Takata, and then variations of this ritual spread throughout the world.

So attunements started their life as a constructed ritual put together by the Imperial Officers, and this ritual has now evolved, changed, altered over time as it has been passed from teacher to teacher in the West. These various attunement methods have been used to attune most of the Reiki people in the world.

So attunements work, of course. They 'connect' the student to Reiki.

Let's make the connection again

But that is not the end of the story: if we are going to get the most out of our Reiki then we are going to have to commit ourselves to working with the energy regularly, on ourselves, on other people, to develop our ability as a channel, to develop our sensitivity to the energy and to develop our intuition. An attunement gives us a baseline connection to the energy, but we can develop ourselves further, and benefit further, through our own efforts.

And in fact we can benefit from receiving further attunements, too. This is something that Reiki Master William Rand has been advocating for many years now, I believe.

He does not say this because attunements are in some way ineffective, or temporary, or weak: he recommends that people get together to re-attune each other because he has found that there are definite benefits associated with having your 'connection' to the energy reinforced or renewed.

So one attunement is enough (or two, or three, or four, or however many attunements you had on your Reiki course, or however many attunements you believe are necessary), but there are definite benefits associated with being reattuned, and if we are serious about our Reiki then we need to also commit ourselves to working with the energy regularly.

You don't just go on a course and that's the end of it: you need to work at your Reiki.

What are Reiju empowerments

When people talk about empowerments, they are referring to **"Reiju empowerments"**.

You can write the word "Reiju" in two different ways using Japanese kanji, one way meaning "accepting the spirituality" and the other meaning "giving the spirituality"; spirituality in this case means 'connection' to the Reiki energy. In fact the word Reiju has been interpreted in several ways, for example "giving of the five blessings" and "the union of mind and ki".

The line in the Reiki precepts where it says "the secret method of inviting happiness through many blessings" might actually mean "the secret method of inviting happiness through receiving many Reiju empowerments".

The empowerments that Mikao Usui used with his students can be referred to as "Reiju" and these were equivalent to a Tendai Buddhist blessing, a blessing that a Tendai teacher would bestow on a student with the intention that the student should receive what they need.

Usui Sensei gave the blessing using intent only, but within Tendai Buddhism there is also a physical ritual that can be carried out which conveys the Reiju blessing; details of this ritual were passed to the West from Usui's surviving students in the late 1990s and it is this ritual that we use on our "Reiki Evolution" First and Second Degree courses.

The effects of empowerments do not wear out

Empowerments 'connect' you to the energy; they allow you to recognise something that is already there.

Just like attunements.

The consensus that I have seen amongst those teachers who are using Reiju in practice, all over the world, is that not only are empowerments effective but they also confer special benefits. In my experience, students who receive Reiju seem 'better connected', better able to work intuitively, more sensitive to the energy in the early stages, when compared with people who have been attuned.

Not everyone will agree with this, but many people who have moved from giving attunements to giving empowerments are saying the same sort of thing.

One empowerment is enough but it is nice do a few on a Reiki course, and we choose to carry out three empowerments on our First and Second Degree courses. But there are definite benefits associated with receiving Reiju repeatedly, and Usui Sensei's students received Reiju from him again and again throughout their training at all levels.

William Rand's recommendation that Masters re-attune each other, because of the benefits associated, serves to echo this original practice. We echo Usui's approach ourselves, by making distant empowerments available for all our students to tune into at any time on a Monday, every week, and Reiju empowerments are also given to students attending our teachers' Reiki shares.

Receiving Reiju regularly helps to 'reinforce' your connection to the source. It enhances self-healing, it helps the student to develop spiritually, it enhances intuition and increases sensitivity to the flow of energy.

Being reattuned will also help to achieve this, though as far as I can see it is not so common within the world of Reiki for re-attunements to be offered.

Now for the nonsense

One or two people are trying to argue that Usui Sensei's method for connecting people to Reiki is ineffective.

They are saying that Reiju is a weak and provides you with only a partial and lowly connection to the energy, that you are actually "dis-empowered", unable to benefit from Reiki properly and unable to treat other people effectively.

These people – who will not have experienced Reiju for themselves, of course, or used Reiju in practice – are also arguing that Reiju-connected students are obliged to desperately carry out energy exercises every day to try and maintain some sort of a decent energy-channelling ability, and that they are dependent on their teacher for a regular 'top' up, without which their Reiki ability will dwindle and disappear.

This is such a distortion of reality!

By way of contrast, they also say that attunements give a far better permanent connection to the source, and the implication is that the student then does not need to carry out any energy work to develop themselves because they are perfectly connected right from the start, and no further commitment or responsibility for personal development is required.

Interestingly, in the same article, I was amused to hear that:

1. You should not treat people with pacemakers. This is nonsense, of course. Please see my article "Restrictions on Reiki" for a longer discussion of this Reiki fable.
2. First Degree does not really give you anything, and you cannot treat yourself and other people effectively at this level. This of course flies in the face of the cumulative experience of hundreds of thousands of people who have taken First Degree and whose lives have changed for the better through Reiki, and who have helped friends and family members at First Degree.
3. You should take Reiki First and Second Degree in one weekend to be able to use Reiki effectively. Again nonsense, and the global consensus is that you should wait between Reiki levels to give yourself a chance to work on yourself and gain confidence, putting what you have learned into practice before moving on. Exhorting people to take Reiki1 and Reiki2 in one go, because they will not be able to do Reiki properly otherwise, is largely a marketing ploy in my view.

Claptrap

There is a lot of nonsense spoken about Reiki, and two more examples that were just sent to me the other day nearly had me choke on my cup of green tea: there is a local college somewhere in the UK (I won't name it) that tells it's Reiki students that they should not treat people who wear contact lenses because the energy will distort the lenses, and in that same part of the country there is also a teacher who is telling their students that every time they use one of the Reiki symbols they are shortening their life by several minutes.

318

We have a word in England for such advice, and for the nonsense that is being written by one or two people about Reiju empowerments: "claptrap".

Claptrap should be avoided at all costs; claptrap will seriously diminish your enjoyment and experience of this wonderful system that we have been given.

So the next time you hear that you shouldn't treat people with pacemakers, or contact lenses, or green trousers for that matter, or the next time you hear that Usui's method of connecting people to the energy doesn't work properly, take such comments with a pinch of salt, ignore them, and move on!

Advice for new Reiki teachers

It's nerve-wracking preparing for your first Reiki course, isn't it? You're taking a step into the unknown and you are going to be guiding a group of people who are trusting you to do a good job. You probably feel that you don't know enough and that you're not ready yet. I know how that feels.

I this article I thought I would just pass on a few pieces of advice that might be of help to you, to ease some of your anxiety. Here goes…

It's OK to teach differently from how you were taught

I'm sure that the First Degree course you went on was great and gave you everything you needed. But the course may be a bit hazy now, given that you have gone on to take Second Degree and your Master Teacher course.

Maybe you have a sense that you would like to do things a bit differently from the way that your teacher taught you: you are a different person, you have a different personality, you approach things in different ways.

And that's ok: you should not feel that you have to exactly replicate the way that they taught or the content of their course. You can be yourself and find your own distinctive way, so long as you pass on the essentials, which you can read about in this article: Back to basics: all about Reiki First Degree. So if you think you can explain things better, provide better course materials, or think the course would flow more logically if you did things differently, go right ahead.

Teach Reiki, not stuff that has nothing to do with Reiki

This is a bit of a bug-bear of mine, but I shall say it anyway: make sure that when you teach Reiki, you just teach Reiki, rather than a whole load of New-Age add-ons that have very little or nothing to do with Usui Reiki but have crept into Reiki over the years, and here I am thinking about smudging, crystal healing, chakra balancing, tarot cards, clairvoyance. When you run a Reiki course I recommend that you teach Reiki, just Reiki.

Make sure that you have practised your attunements well

No matter what lineage you have, you are going to carry out some initiations with your students, whether that be Reiju empowerments or some other variety of attunement ritual. You need to be comfortable in giving these initiations because you don't want to have to keep flicking through your notes half way through the attunements. That would be so unprofessional.

So practise, practise and practise some more! Attune a teddy bear, attune an empty chair, sit in your lounge on a sofa with your eyes closed and imagine in your mind's eye you giving an attunement, see yourself going through the movements, explain out loud what you are doing (as if you were explaining to someone else how to do it), gesticulate so you get used to the hand movements, walk up and down like a mad person, talking yourself through the stages you have learned, draw little stick-figure diagrams to summarise the stages, rap a little rhyme to remind your mind! Be creative!

Once you have the attunements sorted you will feel a lot more confident.

You don't need to have all the answers

You are probably worrying about what people might ask you on your course and whether you will know the answer to all their questions. You probably think that you don't know enough. To be honest, so long as you know more than they do then you will be fine, and you know far more than you think. Your students don't really know anything about Reiki and you have been using it for some time now, so you have a wealth of experience to draw upon.

But there's more to say about questions because you do not have to have the answer to every question; I know I don't. Some questions do not have an answer, or nobody knows, or nobody knows and it doesn't matter anyway. Don't waffle or try to make up an answer: people can tell if you're bullshitting, and if you're honest with your students then they will take more notice of you when you do have something to say.

Remember that Reiki is a practical art

Remember that Reiki is a practical art and that when you teach Reiki you are passing on what you have learned and noticed during your personal experience of working with the energy. You are not passing on high-blown academic theories that you have to revise and might get wrong: you have personal experience of doing all the things that you will be guiding your students through, so you are on very solid ground.

You have given yourself a lot of self-treatments and if you learned Japanese-style Reiki then you will also have experience of using Hatsurei ho most days, and working with the Reiki precepts. You have given Reiki treatments to other people and you have become comfortable with this, learning from your experiences and finding your own comfortable way with the process, making it your own.

You know far, far more about all this stuff than they do, you know far more than you realise, and you have personal experience of doing all the things that you will be guiding your students through... so you can chill, be yourself, and enjoy the day.

And I am sure that you will have a wonderful time on your course.

Structuring your Reiki course

At Reiki Evolution we have a steady stream of students coming to us to re-take their Reiki courses because they weren't very happy with their original Reiki training, and we hear quite a few horror stories about wholly inadequate Reiki training courses.

The main criticisms fall into three categories:

- Aimless drifting through the day of the course, talking about things unrelated to Reiki
- Emerging from the course without a clear idea of what Reiki is or how to use it
- Hardly any hands-on practice at actually doing Reiki, but a lot of talking

So if a student ends up spending their time on a course sipping herb tea while chatting randomly about what everyone thinks of Reflexology or what the last Natural Healing Exhibition everyone went to was like, as if there was no time pressure at all, drifting through the day not really finding out very much about Reiki and not having much of an opportunity to try doing Reiki, that course is not good enough.

Work out your course structure

Effective Reiki courses need to have a definite structure, where the teacher knows in advance what they are going to say, what they are going to demonstrate, what exercises and practices they are going to talk their students through, and what they aim for their students to know and be able to do by the end of the course.

You set a schedule and stick to it because if you spend an hour too much on one particular task or practice then you end up rushing, and skimping, on another area. You need to keep an eye on the time, and stick to your schedule as far as is practical.

Work out what you are going to cover in the morning, and what you are going to cover in the afternoon. Give your students a definite mid-morning break, at a definite time, so you break the morning, and the afternoon for that matter, into two separate sessions, and give your students a definite lunch break; I think lunch should be at least 45 minutes.

Students need a chance to get out of the room, get some fresh air and maybe go for a bit of a walk to clear their heads

In your pre-planned sessions you're there to talk about, demonstrate and supervise people practising Reiki. In your scheduled breaks you can chat about whatever you like, and remember that you need to have a decent break for lunch, too, to clear your head and get some fresh air and a change of scenery.

Reiki Evolution First Degree courses

As an example, here's a list of the 'main headings' from our Reiki First Degree courses:

- Introduction
- Reiju empowerment #1

- Practice: Experiencing energy
- Reiju empowerment #2
- Practice: Daily energy exercises
- Reiju empowerment #3
- Practice: Self-treatments

LUNCH

- Talk/Demo: Treating other people
- Practice: feeling the energy field
- Practice: scanning
- Practice: give and receive a full treatment

You can see that in our morning session, the students receive their three Reiki initiations, they are introduced to the idea of energy and given the chance to feel energy for the first time, they learn how to carry out some daily energy exercises (Hatsurei ho) and they are guided through a form of self-treatment (in this case, the self-treatment meditation that Usui Sensei taught).

The afternoon session moves on from working on yourself to working on other people, with the teacher giving a talk and brief demonstration of a Reiki treatment, showing hand positions, giving hints and tips, and then students practise working with energy again, this time feeling another student's energy field and trying out 'scanning' for the first time. This leads on to the giving and receiving of a full treatment.

Reiki is a practical skill

You will have noticed that there is a lot of hands-on practice in this schedule. There is a good reason for this: Reiki is a practical skill, and you learn a skill by doing it, not just hearing about it. You can't learn to swim by attending lectures about swimming: you have to get in the water and do it, with advice and guidance from your instructor.

It's not enough to tell them what to do: they need to have had practical experience of actually doing the things they will do when using Reiki for themselves and others.

Our aim is for our students to come out of our First Degree course with a clear idea of what Reiki is, where it comes from, and how they can use it simply to work on themselves and treat other people. They will have experienced energy in different ways, practised a self-treatment, used Hatsurei ho and they will have given and received a full Reiki treatment.

These are the essential components of a Reiki First Degree course. You can read more about what Reiki 1 should be about by reading the article entitled "Back to basics: all about Reiki First Degree"

Reiki teaching: explain, guide and review

When you teach someone Reiki, you are teaching a practical skill, an art. Reiki is about things that you do: you meditate, you move energy with visualisation or intention, you move through hand positions as you treat other people, and students need to become comfortable with these practical skills by doing them: initially on their Reiki course and then through repeated practice once they get back home, in the days and weeks after their course.

It occurred to me that when I teach Reiki I go through a particular sequence, with the students sitting in front of me, whenever I teach a particular practice, and you can summarise what I do with these headings:

1. Explain
2. Guide
3. Review

Explain

You need to explain clearly to your students what it is that they will be doing: what the stages are, how they will do it. Maybe you need to demonstrate a few points, or a few movements, and have your students copy you a few times so that they are comfortable with the process, before they do it 'for real'.

Reassure them that they don't need to remember anything at this stage because you will talk them through the process.

Talk about why you do this exercise, what it is said to achieve and what they might notice, reassuring them that everyone is different and that you are not expecting people to experience a particular thing: that there is no 'right' thing that they have to notice.

Guide

Most of the things that we do when we practise Reiki, we do with our eyes closed: meditating, self-treating, performing Hatsurei ho, treating other people, so we need to be guided through these practices for the first time, by a teacher who is paying close attention to us, and who explains what we need to do clearly and carefully, moving everyone through the stages at the same time.

Review

When you have completed an exercise, ask the students what they noticed, what they enjoyed, what they found challenging, how it went for them. You don't necessarily have to go round eliciting feedback in order, say from right to left, because that might be intimidating for the first person you keep on coming to. Just allow the person who feels most comfortable giving their feedback to do so first, but also make sure that you ask everyone what they experienced, so everyone has the chance to share.

It is useful for students to understand that there are differences in their experiences when carrying out a particular exercise and that is ok: everyone is different and experiences things in different ways. And if everyone noticed a particular thing happening, then that's great too!

Feedback is useful because it often raises issues, or questions, that you can use as 'talking points' where you can provide further advice, or practical tips, or talk about perhaps different ways that the exercises can be used (for example, taking Kenyoku out of Hatsurei ho and using it before treating someone).

And if no-one asks the question that would lead you to give that helpful hint or tip, give them the tips anyway.

Explain, Guide, Review, Repeat

You can cycle through these three stages for each chunk of your course: each practical exercise.

So before you give the first attunement or empowerment, explain what you are doing and why, and what they are going to have to do to participate (for example, "bring your hands into the prayer position when I rest my hand gently on your shoulder"), go through the initiation, let them know when you have completed the process for everyone, and get feedback about what people noticed.

When you teach Hatsurei ho, talk about why you do this exercise, the stages they need to go through, the movements that they will need to make (let them practise a few times), guide them through the exercise in real time and then ask for feedback so you can provide useful hints and tips, reassurance, and talk about how the exercise, or parts of the exercise, can be used in different situations.

And so on for self-treatments and treating other people.

On a Second Degree course, for example, you can use the same sequence to introduce meditations on the energies of earth ki and heavenly ki, to deal with distant healing and working intuitively.

Reiki teaching: tell them, tell them and tell them

In my article "Reiki teaching: explain, guide, review" I ran through a simple sequence that you can follow when teaching practical exercises to your students.

In this article I would like to talk about the information that you pass on, how to help the information to stick in your students' minds, and how to ensure that new information relates to what has come before, and is put in proper context.

And in doing this, I will be relying on some very basic advice that is given to people who do public speaking. In fact, this is the most basic public speaking advice!

How to speak in public

When you give a talk to a group of people, you need to:

1. Tell them what you are going to tell them
2. Tell them
3. Tell them what you told them

So you have an introduction where you run over the main themes or areas that you are going to be covering. This starts to give your listeners a 'map of the territory', it provides them with a set of main headings or categories, so when you move on to the next stage ('tell them') you can expand on those themes and headings. The listener already has some 'hooks' in their memory to add the new information to, so it makes sense, has somewhere to fit, and will be more memorable.

Finally, you tell them what you told them, which means that, after having explored the issues in detail, you conclude by bringing them back to the main themes, points, headings that you started with, leaving them with a final summary of your talk. They go away with the main themes clear in their minds.

In doing this, your listeners have received the same information three times, by way of the introduction, by you expanding on these themes in the main part of your talk, and by summarising things at the end. And we know that repeating your exposure to information, particularly when there is some overall structure, where the info relates to a number of clear themes or ideas, and ideally where the information is personally relevant to you or you can imagine how you might use the information in practice, makes that information much more memorable.

So how does this relate to talking to your Reiki students as you progress through their course?

How to make your Reiki course content memorable

Well, you can explain to begin with what is going to be happening during their day, the big items, the main themes or headings. Tell them what they are going to learning about and practising in the morning, and what they will do in the afternoon. I know they will have seen your course schedule in advance but it's a good idea to remind them on the day.

Then, whether you're giving people a quick talk about 'What Reiki is and where it comes from' or 'What Reiki can do for you and the people around you', or whether you are introducing Hatsurei ho or explaining about scanning, you can follow the "tell them, tell them, tell them" sequence: outline the main points, expand on them and then summarise.

Outline, expand, summarise.

Then move on to the next chunk of your day.

Recapping after a break

When you have had a break (your mid-morning break or the lunch break) it is very useful to give them a quick reminder of what they did earlier, summarise the main points very briefly and then move on to the next section, but showing how the next chunk of your day relates to what has come before: how it follows on, how it builds on what they have already done.

You might use a phrase like:

"before the break what we did was to…"

"we learned that…."

"and you discovered that…"

"now we are going to move on by learning about… and practising…"

If you taught Hatsurei ho and had a break, and now you are going to go through self-treatments, you might end up saying something like this (off the top of my head):

"So, before the break we went through Hatsurei ho, a set of daily energy exercises that you can use every day to start to balance your energy system: to clear, cleanse and ground you. You started by using Kenyoku – the dry bathing – where you ritually cleared and cleansed your energy system and then you moved on to move the energy to and from your tanden in time with your breathing, finally focusing the energy on your hands. It doesn't take too long to do, is a wonderful exercise to get into the habit of doing, and the audio CD that came in your study pack talks you through all the stages, so you can relax and just follow the instructions.

"Now we're going to move on to learn how to carry out a self-treatment. There are lots of different ways of doing self-treatments, most of them involving resting your hands on different parts of the body and letting the energy flow. Basically you are firing the energy from lots of different directions to give it the best chance to get to where it needs to go. But sometimes people can find the hand positions a bit awkward or uncomfortable to hold for any amount of time, so fortunately from original Japanese Reiki comes a self-treatment method actually taught by Mikao Usui, where you imagine that the energy is focusing on different areas of your head, and that's what we are going to go through. By treating the head, you actually end up treating the whole body anyway, and it's a lovely routine that you can go through whenever you have the opportunity to close your eyes for a few minutes.

"So, this is what we do..."

PS.

Please do not do this…

By the way, as an aside I wanted to say that you should never read a book or manual out loud to your students.

- It is unprofessional.
- It's so boring: not everyone reads out loud well.
- They can read it themselves so they don't need you to do it for them.

I have heard of courses where most of what happened was the teacher reading out loud to the student from a manual.

This is disgraceful behaviour!

They are there to learn from *you*, not to hear how well you can read out someone else's book.

Never read stuff out to students.

You may as well be a performing parrot.

Reiki teaching: your course materials

Imagine going on a Reiki course, say a First Degree course, for the first time. You don't know anything about Reiki, really, and you're not sure what is going to happen on the course. When you arrive, the teacher starts to tell you huge amounts of information about Reiki during your day. It's difficult to take it all in – it's all so new, after all, and you haven't heard any of this stuff before. There are new ideas and concept to get your head around and you have lots of questions.

You try to take notes as you go along, but it's a bit like trying to drink from a fire hose. You scribble away, and while you're concentrating on what to write down you miss the next bit of what they are saying, and you can hardly replay what they just said! The attunements or empowerments you receive, while often wonderful experiences, don't help either because they have made you feel all spaced out and blissful, and the energy work is zonking you out too, as you try and concentrate on what is being said.

There's a lot to take in.

Then, at the end of the day, you get sent home with a cheery goodbye and two sheets of A4: one with your lineage and one with a bad photocopy of some treatment hand positions.

Reiki students deserve better than that.

So what I am going to talk about in this article are two things that you can do to make sure that your students' experience does not match what I described above.

You can:

- Provide extensive course materials
- Send out course materials to students in advance

Provide extensive course materials

Your students need to relax, safe in the knowledge that everything you say on their Reiki course is covered in detail in their course materials. You should lay out everything that you teach, clearly and logically, with summaries, illustrations or images, and expand on what you teach on the day, providing non-essential but useful information that rounds out and deepens their knowledge of the system that they are learning.

Your students should not be forced to take notes because this is a huge distraction, stops them from enjoying the day, and trying to take decent notes when you're all zonked out on energy is no fun.

So your students deserve a proper course manual that covers *everything* that you dealt with on the course, with further explanations, examples, and back-up info. They should be able to use your manual as a reference work that they can return to again and again to check on everything that is needed for that level.

Give your students variations to experiment with: there is no 'one true way' with Reiki, so suggest different self-treatment methods, and show how they can treat people in different ways, for example short blasts on someone's sore back at work, say, head/shoulder treatments, and full treatments.

Cover everything that you say on a live course, absolutely everything, and more besides, and deal with every question that a student has asked you so that what you provide is really comprehensive: a valuable long-term resource.

Your course materials will be a 'work-in-progress' for some time!

You should also deal with students' learning preferences and make your materials multimedia, and I will talk about this more in a later article.

Send you course materials out in advance

Many years ago when I first started teaching Reiki, I was talking to a Reiki Master that I met at a Reiki gathering or meeting and she mentioned to me that she always sent her students a Reiki manual in advance, before they arrived on the day of their course. My first reaction, because it was different to how I had been taught, was to think, "no, no, no, that's all wrong!" but it didn't take very long before I realised that, actually, that was a genius idea. I wish I could remember her name so I could thank her!

By sending a Reiki manual as soon as a student books on their course, they can take their time and read about Reiki, what it is and where it comes from, what it can do for them, how it can help people you treat, at their leisure. There is no reason why all this information has to be blasted at a student for the first time on the day of a course. They can mull over the information, think about it, search for answers to any questions that they might have, reflect on what they have read.

They will also read about the practical exercises that they are going to be guided through on their live course, so they will already be fairly familiar with Hatsurei ho (daily energy exercises), self-treatments and treating others in different ways.

Info is better assimilated over time, in manageable chunks, rather than trying to 'drink from a fire hose' on the day of a course.

In fact, when I send out study packs to my Reiki Evolution students, I include a couple of audio CDs, a sheet where they can note down their Reiki goals and their initial questions, and I also give them a list of 20 questions that they should be able to answer. I do this so that their subconscious is primed to look for those answers in the course materials, and once they have found the answers then they have focused on the main points or areas that I wanted them to focus on.

By doing this, when they arrive on their live course they are already quite clued-up about Reiki and what they are going to be doing on their live course.

This means that:

1. The teacher does not have to spend their time sitting down telling the students stuff that they could have easily read about beforehand
2. Students can spend most of their time on the live course actually doing stuff with energy rather than

sitting hearing someone talk about, say, the history of Reiki

3. The teacher can spend their time just recapping what the students are already familiar with, focusing the students on the main points and themes and thus reinforcing them

If you're on a live course, it makes sense to make the time you spend count, to make it mostly about experiencing energy and practising using energy on yourself and on other people, rather than just sitting telling students stuff.

Reiki is a practical skill, after all, and rather like riding on a bicycle, you should spend your time practising it, not hearing about it!

Reiki teaching: supporting your students

One of the things that we hear about quite a lot from people who come to Reiki Evolution, having taken a Reiki course before with a different teacher, is that they were never able to get in touch with their previous teacher to ask questions or ask for advice. They felt left out on a limb.

Either the teacher never got back to them, or the student had the impression that the teacher was 'too busy', or the student felt intimidated and didn't want to 'bother' their Reiki teacher.

That's not very good, is it?

So in this article I thought I would talk a bit about the different ways that we can support our students.

Decent course materials and training

The first way that we can help our students to have a great Reiki experience is to make sure that we deal with the common questions that students ask, on our live courses and in our course materials.

When I first started to teach Reiki my students had a lot of questions, and what I did was to remember what a student had asked and make sure that I provided the answer to that question the next time I ran that course, so that over time my courses because more and more helpful, and my course materials because more and more comprehensive.

Over time, I found that the number of questions I received reduced because I was answering them all in advance!

Be happy to help

Make it clear to students that you are happy to answer any questions that they might have, once they have completed their training. Have a state of mind of being friendly, open and supportive and your students will pick up on that.

I tell people that the only stupid question is the question that you do not ask, where you still have this need to have something explained to you, running round your head. That would be the stupid thing!

Now that does not mean that you have to be the source of all Reiki knowledge, on tap, available 24/7. You don't want students asking you questions that are right there in their manual. You can refer them to sources of information, like sections of your manual, or blog posts that you have written, or give them links to web sites etc.

And not all questions are answerable anyway, or the answer might be "who knows?" or "who knows, and it doesn't really matter anyway"

Remember that you are not the source of all Reiki wisdom that your students need to consult for answers about everything: we should not encourage students to be dependent on us as teachers.

You initiate them and they set out on their own journey of discovery and experimentation.

But having said that, you should do what you can to point them in the right direction and keep them focused on the important aspects of Reiki.

Reiki shares

At their most basic, Reiki shares are Reiki get-togethers where you meet other Reiki people and swap Reiki treatments. If there are a fair number of people attending, everyone takes a turn on the treatment table and can end up being treated by multiple practitioners: you might have one person sitting at the head of the table, someone by your ankles and people on either side of the table too.

Receiving a Reiki treatments from lots of people at the same time is an *amazing* experience!

Highly recommended.

Sometimes the Reiki share host (it doesn't have to be a Reiki Master but often is) will talk people though some energy exercises (for example kanyoku followed by Joshin Kokkyu ho) and give attunements (or ideally Reiju empowerments) to everyone present.

If there are several Reiki Masters present, they could 'share out' the empowerments and do a few each. This is ideal if there are new Reiki Masters there who want to practise giving empowerments to people.

Sometimes there might be a further guided meditation or a group distant healing session or a chat about people's experiences when treating other people, say.

You can do what you like.

Set a particular date, say the first Thursday in the month at 7.30pm, or the second Saturday at 2pm, and see what happens.

Reiki practice days

This is a variation on a Reiki share where people have the opportunity to give and receive full Reiki treatments, in pairs, while under the supervision of a Reiki teacher, and is ideal for people who have taken a First Degree course, say, and who haven't had too much of a chance to treat other people, or people who learned Reiki some time ago and now want to get going properly and build their confidence.

The day could again start with some energy exercises and empowerments, and could include a question-and-answer session.

Online support networks

I am a great believer in students providing support to each other, rather than feeling that they have to be dependent on their teacher. Everyone has useful experience that they can share with each other. The Reiki teacher does not know everything, after all.

There are different ways of providing such support, some simpler than others, for example:

A Yahoo! Group

A NING site

A Facebook group

In all these examples, students are able to talk to each other, whether that is through swapping email messages with the whole group (Yahoo!), chatting one-to-one or posting videos and images.

Groups like this can build a tremendous sense of community and you can be sure that if one person posts a question, there will be many other students who were wondering about that too, but didn't ask!

People will share their successes, their amazement, their awe and enthusiasm and the interesting things that have happened to them and to the people they treated. Some will talk about the changes the have noticed within themselves since starting to use Reiki regularly and how they precepts have altered the way they behave and feel about things and changed in the way respond to others.

Highly recommended.

And while to begin with, if you are just starting out as a teacher, you might only have a handful of students subscribed (and tumbleweed blowing through your chat rooms!) it won't be too long before the numbers build up and you'll have on hand a wealth of knowledge and experience that new students can draw upon.

Reiki teaching: what are your goals?

When you are starting to teach Reiki courses and are planning what you are going to cover, demonstrate and say, it is very important that you start with a clear idea of what you're aiming for: your goals.

Goals can encompass what information you want your students to have taken on board and understood, what practical exercises you want them to have been through, and feel comfortable with, and what 'Reiki worldview' you want to instil. I will talk more about this last item further down the page.

Knowledge goals

Most teachers will want their students to have a fairly good idea about:

- What Reiki is
- Where it comes from
- What Reiki can do for them if they work with the energy and the precepts regularly
- What Reiki can do for other people when they receive Reiki treatments

This information can be made available on a web site, so potential students can find out about these areas even before they book on a course. So, for example, the "About Reiki Healing" page of the Reiki Evolution web site starts with this text:

Reiki is a simple Japanese energy system anyone can learn

- Experience peace of mind and inner calm
- Relieve stress and anxiety
- Bring a sense of balance and wholeness
- Help family and friends
- Explore your spiritual side
- Let go of emotional baggage

Further down the page I include links that people can follow to find out more about a whole range of issues to do with Reiki.

If you have your own web site and would like to be able to refer to these articles, please include a link from your web site to any of these pages. Don't copy and paste the text into your own site, though, because Google won't like that and will penalise your site.

Then the information can be repeated, rewritten or summarised in your course materials (your manual, maybe on an audio CD). You will see in my article "Reiki teaching: your course materials" that I recommend that you send your course materials out to your students in advance so they can take their time and mull over this information, and re-visit it several times before arriving on your course, and this means that they day of your course can involve you just re-capping the main points, rather than trying to tell everyone everything, for the first time, on a course where your students are half-zonked-out on the energy and in the worst position to be able to assimilate new information!

How to work out what to tell them

There is a lot of information out there to do with Reiki and it can be difficult sometimes to see the wood for the trees. What do you tell them? What should you start with?

To get some focus, ask yourself this question for each category of information (what Reiki is, where Reiki comes from, What Reiki can do for you etc):

1. If I could only tell my students five things, what would they be?
2. If I had to blurt out the basic info in a 30 second conversation with someone while travelling in a lift, what would I blurt out?

These questions give you an idea of the priorities, the main themes, and then you can expand on these themes and provide additional supporting info and examples. I talk more about this in my article "Reiki teaching: explain, guide and review".

Practical goals

Here is where you decide what practical exercises you want your students to go through on your course, what they need to feel comfortable with, and what they need to understand about what they are doing.

For a First Degree course you might want to focus on:

- Experiencing energy between your hands and around someone else's hands

- Feeling energy around someone else's head and shoulders
- Carrying out Hatsurei ho
- Performing a self-treatment
- Practising scanning
- Giving a full treatment
- Receiving a full treatment

For a Second Degree course you might want to focus on:

- Experiencing the energy of earth ki
- Experiencing the energy of heavenly ki
- Using these two energies to treat someone
- Sending distant healing
- Practising working intuitively
- Exploring use power of intent through visualisation

For each of these, decide what you want them to do, precisely, and how you are going to explain and talk people through these exercises? Work out what you need to the student to understand about what they did. What do these exercises mean for them, why are they important, how will they use them in practice and what might they notice when they carry out these exercises in the coming weeks and months?

More 'global' goals

In a wider sense, my goal is to create independent Reiki practitioners who are comfortable working with the energy, flexible and intuitive in their approach, not attached to dogma, not judgmental of other people's different ways of practising Reiki, and not dependent on me as a teacher to dispense all the answers.

I hope that they should be able to embrace uncertainty, following a Reiki path as a journey of self-development, not believing that what they were taught is the 'one true way' or the 'absolute truth'.

In my article "My Manifesto for Reiki Tolerance" I spoke about how Reiki is a very flexible and accommodating system and acts as a 'carrier' that accommodates very many different ways of working, some simple, some more complex. I spoke about how some ways of working naturally attract some people, while for others a different way of working feels more 'right' for them.

I hope that my students will not treat the Reiki Evolution approach as 'the one true way' and look down on or disparage other practitioners' methods, even though it is not uncommon for some Reiki people to behave in this way.

I want to promote tolerance and respect and compassion for others and I believe that they way that I and my team of teachers speak about Reiki promotes this.

Reiki teaching: using learning preferences

People learn in different ways. When we learn we take in information through our senses, so we see things, we hear things, we learn through doing and we mull things over in our mind. The best learning comes when you provide people with training that engages with all these aspects.

Some people tend to prefer one approach over the others, so you might find that one person much prefers to listen, whereas another might really need to see something before they 'get it', while yet others need to do practical things, to move, to really understand and remember what they are being presented with.

In NLP (Neurolinguistic Programming) these preferences are called being visual, or auditory or kinaesthetic. There is another preference, too, when people are referred to as 'audio digital': these people need a strong sense of order or logic before things sink in properly for them.

I am quite a visual person, so I like diagrams, I think in pictures (not everyone does), I use Mind Maps, my written notes are quite visually diverse and sometimes flamboyant. I need that visual input more than, say, listening to something. And I have a great need for logic and order.

"The SatNav episode"

This was brought home to me several years ago when I was training in NLP and my wife Lorraine and I were going somewhere fairly local that we had not been to before.

We had the SatNav on but hadn't bothered to attach it to the windscreen; Lorraine had it resting in her lap and she looked at it and told me where to go.

Lorraine prefers the auditory sense so it made sense to her to just call out the instructions to me on this fiddly route; she said that I didn't need to see the screen. I thought that I didn't... But I did! I really did! It was excruciating for me to travel without seeing a map of where I was going.

I had to stop the car in the end and look at the SatNav screen so I could *see* where I was. Once I had seen the territory it all made sense and I understood where I needed to go.

I needed to see to understand, whereas Lorraine didn't have that need.

When I give directions to someone I always want to reach for a scrap of paper so I can show someone; they might respond, though, by saying "just tell me!" My mind will be saying, "it's much better if I can show you."

But for them it may not be...

Don't assume everyone is just like you

The problem comes because we tend to assume that the way we learn is they way that everybody learns. So if you learn by listening, you might run a course where you spend most of your time talking, and there will be students who are desperate to see something demonstrated, or to see a diagram, or to have an overview of what they day will entail, or to see the logical links between things, or to try something out for themselves, to 'get their hands dirty'.

So by running a course where you show things, you talk about things, you supervise people practising stuff, and you make sure that your day flows logically from one thing to another, you are providing your students with the very best training.

You are touching all bases and making sure that the course meets the learning preferences of all your students.

And by touching all bases, you actually make the learning more meaningful and effective for everyone, because the best learning uses sights, sounds and physicality, no matter what someone's preference might be. So a 'visual' learner like me needs images, but I will learn better if I also get to hear and to do.

Making your courses touch all bases

- On a live course it is straightforward to make sure that you are touching all bases: On a First Degree course, for example:
- Talk to them about Reiki and about the exercises they will be carrying out
- Show them what they will be doing when they perform the movements of Hatsurei ho and a Self-treatment
- Have them go through the physical movements with you

- Make sure they have seen you make the movements and practised the physical movements for themselves before they close their eyes for you to guide them with your voice

When dealing with the subject of treating other people, you can talk about the subject and then you can give a visual demonstration of the hand positions, talking to your students when you do that to give hints and tips and useful advice. They then go through the hand positions themselves, guided by your voice.

Teaching materials to use on the day

You might consider having some display boards set up, with colour photographs demonstrating full treatment hand positions. Your students will take the information in subconsciously during the day.

On my Reiki Master Teacher live courses I used to have display boards set up which showed the stages of giving Western-style attunements. They can see the visuals as you talk them through the process, then you give them a visual demonstration, then they go through the movements themselves with you or another student talking them through the stages.

I even had some A3 sheets and marker pens so students could draw little diagrams to explain the attunement stages, and I also had students sit down and talk each other through the process.

So I was engaging with all senses: they looked and were were watching, they listened and they explained; it is very powerful having someone explain something to another person because you have to have things well-ordered in your mind in order to do that. They created visuals and they carried out physical movements while receiving spoken instructions.

All in all, a powerful learning combination.

Creating course materials that engage all senses

At Reiki Evolution we use detailed and comprehensive course manuals containing text, summaries and photographs. The manuals are well ordered and logical and students get to read about the experiences of many other students that have been through this training.

Along with the printed manual, students for First Degree also receive separate "at a glance" summary sheets with lots of photographs to illustrate the stages of carrying out Hatsurei ho, giving a Self-treatment, and some Full treatment hand positions.

I include some blank 'cartoon strip'-style squares for them to do little drawings, perhaps just with stick figures, to illustrate the treatment hand positions, to jog their memory. I also include a set of "20 Reiki questions", the answers to which they are expected to search for in their course materials, and I include a separate sheet with the answers that they can look at to check their discoveries.

We provide audio CDs with commentary (just like listening to a Reiki training course, but something that you can play again and again) and we also provide guided meditations, talking students through their daily energy exercises, a self-treatment meditation, a distant healing meditation and a Reiki symbol meditation.

You can see why we do that, can't you? We provide logic and order, we provide written information, summaries and images, we provide short talks you can listen to and we give you the chance to be guided as you put Reiki into practice on yourself and with other people.

Engaging with people's different learning preferences, and ensuring that your live course and your training materials are multimedia, leads to the most powerful and effective learning.

Reiki teaching: using the right 4MAT

That is not a spelling mistake: I did intend to spell the word 'format' in that way! The "4MAT" system is a way of approaching teaching that was created by Bernice McCarthy and proposes that there are four major learning styles, each of which result in a student asking different questions and displaying different strengths during the learning process.

The 4MAT system is based on Myers-Briggs personality typing, which break people down into different categories, for example Introvert and Extrovert.

I am not going to go into detail here about the different categories (you can read up about those for yourself if you're interested) but beyond Introvert/Extrovert there are three other pairs of categories:

Sensor/Intuitor
Thinker/Feeler
Judger/Perceiver

Myers Briggs uses these labels to create four-letter abbreviations for particular personality types, so someone might be an "INFJ", an Introvert, Intuitor, Feeler, Judger. Myers Briggs aficionados will know immediately what sort of a person that is!

But let's get back to teaching and Reiki...

The four 4MAT categories

The 4MAT system describes four different types of learners, all of whom require different things in order to best assimilate information. Here are the four types:

The Concrete-Random learner

This learner needs to know "**Why?**" they are learning a particular thing, why they should be involved in a particular activity. What is the point of all this?

The Abstract-Sequential learner

This learner needs to know "**What?**" to learn: exactly what do they need to know? They need to see it in black and white; it shouldn't be vague and wishy-washy. There shouldn't be unanswered questions.

The Concrete-Sequential learner

This learner wants to know "**How?**" to apply the information they are being presented with: what do you actually do with this information in practice?

The Abstract-Random learner

This learner wants to answer "**What If?**" questions about how they can modify what they have learned to make it work for them.

Using 4MAT in practice

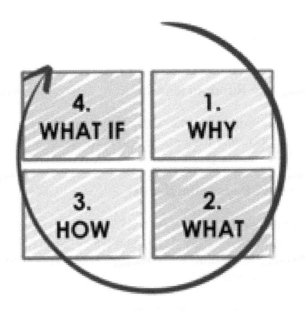

You can use the four questions – Why?, What?, How? and What If? to guide you when teaching a course or teaching a particular technique or practice.

If you deal with these four different questions, you make the learning accessible to the four major categories of learners, make what you teach memorable and ensure that you leave no-one behind.

These four questions can be cycled through again and again for each section of your course. Let's think of an example: say, the teaching of Hatsurei ho (daily energy exercises used in Japanese-style Reiki). This is how the teaching of it, 4MAT-style, might look like:

Hatsurei ho teaching, 4MAT-style

Why do we do Hatsurei ho? What is the purpose of it and what are our goals in carrying it out?

What do we actually do when we perform Hatsurei ho? What are the stages, what precisely will we do in what order? What do we need to know in order to perform Hatsurei ho effectively?

How do we do Hatsurei ho? This would be a good time to talk your students through the process and talk about when to do Hatsurei ho, how often, and what happens if you miss a day.

Finally, how can you modify Hatsurei ho and use it in different contexts? This is the "**What If**?" stage: you might talk about separating out Kenyoku and using it for cleansing/clearing prior to starting a Reiki treatment, or in other situations. You might also talk about using just Kenyoku and Joshin Kokkyu ho, a shorter sequence which comes closer to what Usui Sensei was teaching to his students in Japan.

That's not a bad sequence to keep cycling through, is it?

You can introduce a topic or exercise by explaining why you would want to go through this exercise, you move on to explain in detail exactly what the exercise is, you describe how the exercise is used in practice and then finish by exploring different ways in which the exercise can be used, in different contexts and situations.

So you can see that the 4MAT system provides you with a way of being comprehensive with your teaching of each chunk of your course, while meeting the learning needs of all your students.

Over to you

Why not look at the different things that you teach on your Reiki courses, and see how well your presentations, descriptions and demonstrations meet these four learning criteria.

How could you alter what you say and do to follow the 4MAT system in these examples?

- Self-treatments
- Head/shoulder treatments
- Distant healing
- Using the Reiki symbols
- Working intuitively

How Reiki Evolution can help you with your Reiki courses

Did you know that people all over the world are using Reiki Evolution course manuals and audio CDs on their Reiki courses? And not just people who have trained with Reiki Evolution: people from all Reiki lineages and styles.

The reason for that is that I seem to have put together some resources that aren't available anywhere else (from what I have seen):

Reiki manuals

I have created professionally printed and bound course manuals that are detailed, comprehensive and easy to read, containing careful descriptions, images and summaries that make it easy for students to get to grips with all the main practices of Reiki healing.

I have manuals for you to use as follows (all A4 size):

- Reiki First Degree (Shoden) – 170 pages
- Reiki Second Degree (Okuden) – 110 pages
- Reiki Master Teacher (Shinpiden) – 230 pages

Read what Sherry Coffman, a Reiki Master Teacher from Texas, USA, thinks about Reiki Evolution course manuals:

"When I first started my journey with Reiki, I was not provided with a manual of any kind. I was given a resource list and a folder with some handouts. My original Reiki Master Teacher was unable to complete the Master level training with me due to personal illness and so I had to move on to another Master Teacher.

It turned out to be the best thing that could have happened for me because the new Master was using Taggart King's manuals. So, I was introduced to the materials with Shinpiden. When I decided to begin conducting my own trainings, I reviewed First Degree with my new Master. That's when I saw the Shoden manual for the first time. At that point I was hooked and now I provide the appropriate level manual for my students as part of their training.

"Using Taggart's manuals fits my personality as a teacher. They are direct, complete and give full explanations with visuals for anything that a blooming practitioner could need. I especially love his sense of humor and the way he brings a reality to every day Reiki while still holding a space of total respect for the wisdom and mystery of Reiki. He speaks with the voice of authority, but encourages students to be guided by personal intuition. I especially appreciate his commitment to researching and sharing the original Japanese ways, making it clear where and how Western Reiki traditions have entered the scene.

"Using his materials gives me confidence as a teacher knowing my students have a quality manual to which they can refer in the days following their training."

Reiki audio CDs

You will have seen from the various articles that I have written that I believe it is important to provide students with course materials that meet their different learning styles, and how important it is to provide comprehensive training materials that students can revisit after their training day.

Reiki audio CDs help with this a great deal because they can listen to a potted version of a Reiki course – hearing the main points of what they would hear on a live training day – and also be guided through the main energy exercises and meditations and self-treatments that we teach.

So I have audio CDs for you that either provide commentary (like listening to a live course) or guided meditations:

- Reiki First Degree commentary
- Reiki Second Degree commentary
- "Reiki Meditations" (suitable for First and Second Degree and consists of: Hatsurei ho, Self-treatment meditation, Symbol meditation and Distant healing session)
- "Talking you through a Reiki treatment" – does what it says on the tin! – talks you through a full, hour-long Reiki treatment.
- Reiki Master Teacher commentary
- Reiki Master Teacher guided instructions (talks you through a Reiki attunement, a Japanese Reiju empowerment, a session where you open to intuition (the Japanese 'Reiji ho' method) and a special 'Frequency scale' meditation that Taggart devised

Reiki Certificate templates

I know that one of the things that can be quite challenging to begin with, when you start running your own Reiki courses, is to get together decent-looking Reiki certificates.

To help people with this I enlisted the help of a Japanese Calligraphy Master, who has brushed for me a traditional Japanese certificate, using Japanese calligraphy, that can be used for any Reiki course or training.

I have put together Reiki certificate templates that you can download or order on DVD-rom. They come in different formats and with all the special kanji that you would need to create gorgeous Japanese-style certificates for your students.

See what some Reiki Masters thought of the Reiki certificate templates:

"I have now used the CD Rom that you supplied to me for making Reiki Certificates. I have used it on two occasions and found it easy to use and the end result is good and looks very professional. I liked the fact that I could choose different wordings re attunements, empowerments, initiations. Thank you for making this available: without it I would, no doubt, be floundering around wondering how to do it!"

Sally Beautista, London

"I used the Reiki Certificates CD-ROM for a Reiki 1 course last weekend, which I ran on a one/one for a lady who wanted to learn Reiki to use on her farm animals. Not being 'into' computers apart from emails etc. I was very pleased with the certificate I produced with your CD."

Geraldine Shuttleworth, Staffordshire

"The Certificates CD I received was extremely good value for money. I did make some amendments to personalise my certificates as you suggested. Another fantastic resource with step by step instructions for the technophobes amongst us (I am referring to myself of course!). Anyone that has any of your other CD's will know how the energy flows when they are played and this resource CD is no different. It set my creative side alight! I was instinctively drawn to the CD and you did not disappoint."

Caron Sanders-Crook, London

I am very pleased with the CD-ROM it has been very useful to have a template, especially a choice of templates to work with. I am not that computer literate so it was nice to be able to produce something that looks so professional."

Rachel Robinson, West Midlands

Discounts for ordering resources in 'multipacks'

I have put together packs of 4 Reiki manuals or CDs that you can order at reduced prices.

I have priced the packs so that you receive a discount of 33% compared with retail price (First Degree manual) and a discount of 50% for the audio CDs.

When you order the Reiki manuals, I arrange for them to be specially printed for you and they go in the post to you in a couple of days, whether that's in the UK, USA, Canada, Australia, or anywhere else in the world.

I post you your audio CDs the next working day, and they are mainly ordered by UK Reiki teachers.

Here is the web page where you can order discounted packs of books and manuals:

http://www.reiki-evolution.co.uk/buying-in-bulk/

Below you can read some comments from other Reiki Masters who are using Reiki Evolution course materials:

"I have used Reiki Evolution course materials for some time. It is a pleasure to use them as they are clear and comprehensive, easy to follow with clear diagrams and instructions.

"All materials are produced to a high specification – creating an image of professionalism. The manuals are a good reference for students to browse through, enabling them to reflect and digest all that has been given and shown to them.

"The CDs too, assist with all aspects covered including meditations. For those students with dyslexia the CDs have proved very popular."

Oonagh Van Hemuss, Reiki Master Teacher

"I have been using Reiki Evolution resources ever since I started running my own courses and teaching Reiki. This is mainly because I don't believe in re-inventing wheels! There is such depth of information in the manuals, even if I wanted to, I could not produce anything better myself.

"From a personal point of view, I return to the manuals time and time again to refresh my knowledge and check what I may have overlooked. I really like the fact that within the manuals there are options and little is set in stone. I can choose for myself which approaches to take both when self treating and when giving a Reiki treatment so I can choose the techniques which work best for me. Re-visiting the manuals gives me the opportunity to find techniques I've left aside and try them when I'm ready to. This is very much the approach I suggest to all my Reiki students.

"There is always positive feedback from people on my Reiki courses about both the manuals and the CDs. As a teacher of Reiki, it is great having such excellent resources readily available to distribute.

"People who book on my courses have often trained to level 1 or 2 with another Reiki lineage so I always ask to see any manuals or support materials they have been given. This allows me to see the similarities across the courses and

where I might wish to include additional elements on the course.

Whilst there are some good support materials out there, to date, no other manual has come close to the depth of the manuals provided by Reiki Evolution. In fact, in many cases there have been no support materials or 'manuals' that consist of around 10 pages of large font containing only a small amount of information. With the Reiki Evolution manual there is no need to flounder after the course and struggle to remember everything as it can be referred to time and time again.

"In my experience, very few other lineages distribute CDs as part of their courses. Reiki Evolution CDs are a great aid to learning and back up information in each manual. They can be played in the background or in the car until all of the information is absorbed, or used in a more structured way as the pre-course study course is followed. The CDs also serve as a good refresher after the course.

"The meditation CDs are excellent and help to quickly get the listener relaxed and reach a meditative state…backed up by endless comments from my Reiki students about how much they love Taggart's voice. Occasionally I get approached by previous students who have not given Reiki much attention for a while – the meditation CD can help people to find their way back to Reiki.

"Many people, years after they have completed their Reiki courses tell me they still use the meditation CD regularly…it's easy, it works so why not?

Rhonda Bailey, Reiki Master Teacher